Contents

About the Authors

Mary A. Fristad, Ph.D.

Dr. Mary A. Fristad is a 1986 graduate of the University of Kansas clinical psychology program. She completed her clinical child psychology internship at Brown University and is board certified in clinical psychology. She is an Associate Professor of Psychiatry and Psychology at the Ohio State University, where she has been on faculty since 1986. Dr. Fristad is the Director of Research and Psychological Services in the Ohio State University Division of Child and Adolescent Psychiatry. She supervises and provides general assessment and treatment services to the inpatient, day treatment, and outpatient programs. She directs the child psychometric laboratory, where children and adolescents can be assessed for mental retardation, learning disabilities, other learning difficulties, and giftedness, as well as functioning in the home and school settings. Her area of specialty is childhood mood disorders. Dr. Fristad has served on NIMH review committees; sits on the American Psychological Association Task Force for Serious Mental Illness; has been the principal and coprincipal investigator on over a dozen federal, state, local grants; and is the author of more than 50 scientific articles.

Marijo Teare Rooney, Ph.D.

Dr. Marijo Teare Rooney is a 1991 graduate of the University of Louisville clinical psychology program. She completed a clinical psychology internship at Topeka State Hospital and a postdoctoral fellowship in child psychology at the University of Kansas School of Medicine–Wichita. She is a member and serves as Secretary of the Kansas Psychological Association. She actively promotes its agenda at the state legislative level. Dr. Teare Rooney is currently in private practice.

Elizabeth B. Weller, M.D.

Elizabeth Weller, M.D., graduated from the American University in Beirut in 1975 after a pediatric internship. She completed her psychiatry residency at Washington University in St. Louis and her training in child and adolescent psychiatry at the University of Kansas Medical Center. Dr. Weller currently is Professor of Psychiatry and Pediatrics and Vice Chair of the Department of Psychiatry at the University of Pennsylvania School of Medicine. Previously, she held faculty appointments at the University of Kansas and The Ohio State University. On the national level, Dr. Weller has served as President of the Society of Biological Psychiatry; as a member of the Executive Council of the American Association of Directors of Residency Training; as a council member and Program Director of the American Association of Clinical Psychiatrists; and as a council member of the American Academy of Child and Adolescent Psychiatry. She is currently a director of the American Board of Psychiatry and Neurology.
Dr. Weller has conducted research and published extensively in the area of mood disorders and bereavement in children and adolescents. She and her spouse, Dr. Ronald A. Weller, have received federal, state, and local research grants to support their studies.

Ronald A. Weller, M.D.

Dr. Ronald A. Weller is a graduate of the Washington University School of Medicine. He completed a psychiatry residency at Barnes and Renard Hospital in St. Louis, Missouri. Dr. Weller is currently on the faculty at the University of Pennsylvania in Philadelphia. Previously, he held faculty appointments at the University of Kansas and The Ohio State University, where he was Director of Residency Education and Training. He is active in many professional organizations and is a past president of The American Academy of Clinical Psychiatrists. He has also been an active researcher and has published approximately 100 scientific articles and book chapters.

Preface

The Children's Interview for Psychiatric Syndromes (ChIPS) began as an idea in the Division of Child Psychiatry at the University of Kansas School of Medicine. We were interested in developing a diagnostic interview for children that employed strict DSM-III (American Psychiatric Association 1980) criteria and was brief, succinct, and simple to administer. Our team had used and helped develop structured diagnostic interviews for adults (i.e., the Psychiatric Diagnostic Interview [PDI; Othmer et al. 1981]) and children (i.e., the Diagnostic Interview for Children and Adolescents [DICA; Herjanic and Reich 1982]). Thus, we were familiar with structured interviewing as a method of assessment. We became interested in developing a new, streamlined children's interview from the ground up rather than trying to modify an existing interview.

Our efforts produced an interview that has since been modified for DSM-III-R and DSM-IV (American Psychiatric Association 1987 and 1994, respectively). The technical studies and reports from frequent users indicate that our efforts were successful. Reliability and validity of the ChIPS have been established. Those who use the ChIPS like its ease and brevity of administration.

The ChIPS, like any structured interview, is not intended to replace the clinician. It is, however, a quick and efficient method of gathering information that can then be used by a clinician to provide a more cost-effective and comprehensive clinical interview.

We wish to acknowledge the following individuals and institutions, who facilitated the completion of our studies using the ChIPS:

- The study interviewers: Gabrielle Aponte; Carol Bolt, M.A.; Jim Cummins, B.S.; Alissa Glickman, B.S.; Louise Kimmel, B.A.; Michael McCreight, B.A.; Anita Misra, B.S.; Mary Jo Petrosky, B.A.; Mohammed Shafii, M.D.; Heather Spence, B.S.; Carolyn Spohn, R.N.; Alison Tait, B.A.; and Joe Zubosky, B.S.

- Quinn Chipley, M.A., who coordinated the Louisville interview team and also completed study interviews

- Jim Cummins, B.S., and Alissa Glickman, B.S., who assisted in preparing the case reports for this manual based on interviews they conducted

- Paul Salmon, Ph.D., who chaired Dr. Teare Rooney's master's thesis and dissertation committees at the University of Louisville

- Barbara Burns, Ph.D., Elton Quinton, Ph.D., Joe Aponte, Ph.D., Samuel Himmelfarb, Ph.D., and Edward Hampe, Ph.D., who served on Dr. Teare Rooney's master's thesis and/or dissertation committees

- Joseph S. Verducci, Ph.D., who provided statistical consultation for this project

- Nicole Demers, M.S., who assisted in data management and analysis

- The staffs at the Bingham Child Guidance Clinic and the Ackerley Psychiatric Unit in Louisville, Kentucky; the child psychiatry inpatient unit at the University of Kansas Medical Center, Kansas City, Kansas; and the Child and Adolescent Outpatient Clinic and child inpatient unit at Ohio State University, Columbus, Ohio

Chapter 1: Introduction

Description of the ChIPS

The ChIPS is designed for use with children ages 6 to 18 years. It is based on strict DSM-IV criteria and is appropriate for clinical and research use. The ChIPS screens for the presence of the following 20 disorders:

- Attention-Deficit/Hyperactivity Disorder
- Oppositional Defiant Disorder
- Conduct Disorder
- Substance Abuse
- Specific Phobia
- Social Phobia
- Separation Anxiety Disorder
- Generalized Anxiety Disorder
- Obsessive-Compulsive Disorder
- Acute Stress Disorder
- Posttraumatic Stress Disorder
- Anorexia
- Bulimia
- Depressive Episode
- Dysthymic Disorder
- Manic Episode
- Hypomanic Episode
- Enuresis
- Encopresis
- Schizophrenia/Psychosis

In addition, the ChIPS inquires about psychosocial stressors, including child abuse/neglect. Each section of the interview that reviews disorders consists of a series of questions pertaining to the DSM-IV diagnostic criteria for that particular disorder. The interview has been constructed so that affirmative answers indicate pathology. For each disorder, questions have been organized in a "branching" format. The first several questions function as screening questions for the disorder, because the symptoms they address are frequently endorsed by children with that disorder. After these questions are asked, the interview may "branch" in one of two ways. If a child's response to the screening questions is not positive, the interviewer may skip the remaining questions in that section and continue with the next disorder. If a child answers in the affirmative (thereby indicating possible pathology), the remaining questions in the section are asked. After all questions pertaining to symptoms for a disorder have been asked, questions about symptom onset and duration, as well as about impairment resulting from the symptoms, are asked. Finally, for some disorders, a type or subtype is recorded (e.g., for Attention-Deficit/Hyperactivity Disorder, whether the symptoms are predominantly Inattentive, Hyperactive–Impulsive, or Combined).

The ChIPS is a highly structured interview. Questions are designed to be asked word for word, and examples of alternative phrasings are provided.

> *Example from Attention-Deficit/Hyperactivity Disorder section:*
>
> 2. a) **Do you have trouble staying in your seat (for example, in school or at the dinner table)?**

Here some explanatory examples are provided in parentheses. If the interviewer needs to provide further clarification, "Can you stay in your chair in school?" or some other similar rephrasing may be used.

The conditions necessary for meeting DSM-IV criteria for a disorder are also completely specified on the scoring form that accompanies the interview. Although it may superficially appear that this method leaves nothing to chance, areas exist in which the interviewer can err and thus lower the validity of the interview. Three categories of errors are branching-format errors, comprehension errors, and elaboration errors. A discussion of these errors appears in Chapter 7 of this manual.

Principles of Use

Population. Although the ChIPS was originally designed for use with children 6 to 12 years of age, its age range was subsequently expanded to include adolescents (13 to 18 years of age). The ChIPS initially focused on younger children to ensure that the language used was appropriate for that population. When the age expansion occurred, the language of the instrument was not changed. While there was concern that the simple language might offend teenagers, this concern appears to have been unwarranted. Because the interview relies on the active participation of the child or adolescent, adequate receptive and expressive language abilities are a prerequisite. ChIPS validation studies have been conducted only in English-speaking populations, and the demographic distribution of the study samples was largely Caucasian. Test users should be sensitive to possible cultural and ethnic differences when interpreting test results.

Interviewer qualifications. The ChIPS is designed to be administered by trained lay interviewers. A clinician should oversee the training in and administration of this instrument and should be responsible for the interpretation of its results.

Training. Chapter 7 of this manual outlines five specific steps to be followed in training interviewers to conduct ChIPS interviews that are both reliable and valid. These steps should be completed under the guidance of a clinician who is familiar with DSM-IV, child and adolescent psychopathology, and the format of structured diagnostic interviews and, ideally, who has undergone similar training in ChIPS administration. These steps are briefly described below.

The first step, *familiarization*, involves reading and studying the interview and the manual and reviewing pertinent sections of DSM-IV to develop an awareness of childhood psychopathological conditions. Step 2, *review of general interviewing procedures*, acquaints trainees with common problem areas and general concerns about diagnostic interviewing. *Review of specific disorders*, the third step, focuses on the specific syndromes covered in the ChIPS and the details of particular questions in each section. The fourth step, *observation of live interviews and videotapes*, provides trainees with a standardized demonstration of interview techniques and affords an opportunity to practice scoring the ChIPS. Finally, step 5, *supervised in vivo practice*, ensures that trainees are equipped to meet the challenges of actual ChIPS administration.

Limitations of the instrument. The ChIPS was designed to identify the symptoms of 20 common Axis I psychiatric disorders in children and adolescents. It does not consider other DSM-IV conditions or diagnoses. It is not designed to detect mental retardation or learning disorders. It is not a measure of personality. Because of the ChIPS' self-report format, the information obtained is only as reliable as the informant from whom it comes. Thus, it is inappropriate to administer the ChIPS to anyone who is clearly unable (e.g., due to active psychosis) or unwilling (e.g., due to a general reluctance to cooperate with mental health professionals) to provide accurate information. If the ChIPS is administered to such a person, the clinician interpreting the results must bear in mind the limitations of information elicited under such circumstances (for a more detailed discussion, refer to Chapter 6 of this manual). The ChIPS is a screening instrument. As such, its questions are designed to over- rather than underidentify potential problem areas. Thus, all symptoms, even those of insufficient number or severity to meet diagnostic criteria, are brought to the attention of a clinician, who can then decide how they fit within the overall clinical picture.

Ethical standards. Ethical standards as they apply to testing (*Standards for Educational and Psychological Testing* [American Psychological Association 1985]) also apply to the ChIPS. The ChIPS should be administered after voluntary and informed consent has been obtained from the child's parent(s). It is also important to obtain assent from the child. When the ChIPS is administered in a clinical setting, verbal assent suffices. In a research setting, however, written assent should be obtained. Because the ChIPS becomes part of the child's clinical record, results should be treated as confidential.

Appropriate settings.   The ChIPS can be used in any setting in which psychiatric diagnoses are desired. This includes inpatient units, outpatient facilities, training centers, and research environments. In clinical settings, the ChIPS can be used as a screening interview to maximize the efficiency of the clinician's time.

Chapter 2: Theoretical Foundations

History of Child Assessment

The field of child psychodiagnostics has its roots in the field of adult psychopathology. In the psychoanalytic tradition of Sigmund Freud, childhood was considered important only from the perspective of its influence on the mature adult (Kessler 1971). Anna Freud and Erik Erikson expanded this narrow concentration by advocating investigation of child psychopathology for the child's sake (Kessler 1971; Maier 1965). This new viewpoint served to refocus the field's attention from the adult to the child.

By emphasizing the observable behaviors of the child (Kessler 1971; Maier 1965), Jean Piaget and John Watson brought a more objective outlook to the field. Watson further expanded the field of childhood psychopathology by providing a framework of treatment with his "Habit Clinics" (Kessler 1971). The Child Guidance Movement led to additional refinement of child diagnostics and treatment. By considering the child's behavior and environment, a more complete diagnostic formulation could be obtained (Stevenson and Smith 1934).

The establishment of objective criteria for the investigation of child psychopathology in the population as a whole is the most recent step in the evolution of child psychodiagnostics. Although it attempts to be atheoretical, this epidemiological/empirical approach to child assessment is largely based on the medical model (see review by Cantwell 1988) and is primarily concerned with classification of disorders within a reliable and valid framework. Many factors (e.g., environmental, developmental, psychoanalytic, physiological) can influence behavior, and a behavior's etiology cannot always be determined through observation. Thus, psychodiagnostics began to move away from etiological diagnoses and toward a broader assessment of functioning (see review by Kessler 1971). The goal was to base the classification of disorders on factual information as much as possible, and not on a particular theoretical framework. Such a classification system would be able to differentiate between the categories in the system and also to distinguish between normality and abnormality.

Toward this end, a diagnostic classification scheme—the Diagnostic and Statistical Manual (DSM)—was created by the American Psychiatric Association in 1952. Since this first version, subsequent revisions have been published (American Psychiatric Association 1968, 1980, 1987, 1994), the most recent of which is DSM-IV. The DSM system is the classification scheme used by most clinical and governmental agencies in the United States (American Psychiatric Association 1994).

Development of Structured Interviews

Diagnostic interviews provide a means to increase reliability and precision in the field of diagnostics (Edelbrock and Costello 1984). Such interviews are designed to systematically assess whether specific symptoms and symptom clusters are present for the purpose of identifying disorders (Chambers et al. 1985). These instruments have evolved considerably, moving from open-ended clinical interviews to semistructured interviews and, more recently, to highly structured questionnaires and symptom checklists (Robins 1985). The three basic developments in the evolution of diagnostic interviews are discussed below in their historical contexts.

Stage 1. As development of specific criteria to diagnose child psychopathology has progressed, techniques to assess mental disorders in children have undergone a concurrent evolution. Prior to the introduction of DSM-II (American Psychiatric Association 1968), there were no accepted definitions of symptoms, symptom clusters, or diagnoses for children. Early diagnostic evaluations of children were based primarily on information gleaned from parents and from "play session" interviews with the child. The first standardized interview for assessing children was developed by Lapouse and Monk (1958). This interview schedule used the mother as the primary informant; the child was not interviewed. The goal of Lapouse and Monk's interview was to provide a descriptive picture of the child's behavior. Because the authors knew that sampling only the mother's perspective of the child's behavior might result in incomplete information, they used separate surveys of the mother and the child to establish the reliability of their interview (Lapouse and Monk 1958).

Stage 2. Efforts were then initiated to find ways of eliciting information directly from the child. Rutter and Graham (1968) developed a semistructured clinical interview schedule for children. They, and others since (Costello et al. 1982; Herjanic et al. 1975; Hodges et al. 1982; Kovacs 1985; Puig-Antich and Chambers 1978), have demonstrated that symptom-oriented interviews of children are a reliable way to obtain diagnostic information.

Stage 3. As clinicians and researchers became more adept at directly interviewing children, it was recognized that parents often were not sufficiently aware of their children's inner life to accurately report their thoughts and emotions. Edelbrock and colleagues (1986) demonstrated that a higher level of agreement between parent and child interviews occurred when the instruments focused on objective and easily observable symptoms. Moreover, behavioral observations were deemed unsatisfactory in evaluating "intrapsychic" symptoms (Chambers et al. 1985). Because the reliability of children's interviews has now been demonstrated, assessment of childhood disorders has progressed to the point where the direct interview of a child is an integral part of the assessment process.

Current Status of Structured Interviews

Just as advances in DSM-III, DSM-III-R, and DSM-IV have resulted in decreased variance in criteria used to make particular diagnoses, the use of diagnostic interviews has reduced the uncertainty about what information has actually been collected from a child. A variety of assessment instruments have been developed for childhood disorders, ranging from open-ended diagnostic interviews to more structured interviews and symptom checklists (Chambers et al. 1985; Edelbrock and Costello 1984). Structured interviews consist of specific questions to be asked, explicit criteria for assessing responses, and detailed instructions for conducting the interview and recording the results. There are two types of structured interviews: highly structured and semistructured. Each has unique advantages, as reviewed below.

Advantages of highly structured interviews.   There are at least six advantages to using highly structured interviews. First, because lay interviewers and research technicians can be trained to use them, these interviews provide a relatively low-cost method of eliciting important clinical information. Research indicates that highly structured interviews minimize the effects of the interviewer's level of training (Jaynes et al. 1979). Second, these interviews generally take less time to administer than more traditional, indirect methods (Herjanic and Reich 1982). Third, more clinical information can be obtained and recorded during the initial structured interview than is possible during an open-ended interview. Fourth, unlike open-ended interviews, which tend to limit their focus primarily to the presenting problem, structured interviews provide systematic screening of disorders. This approach may lead to the exploration of areas that clinicians might otherwise overlook (Rutter and Graham 1968) and guards against possible biases on the part of the clinician. Thus, the reliability of psychiatric diagnoses may be increased by routinely examining areas other than the obvious presenting problem (Helzer 1981). Fifth, structured interviews provide an additional source of information in the comprehensive assessment of child psychopathology, as they allow children to report symptomatology from their own point of view. Sixth, given the recent increase in emphasis by managed mental health care companies on standardized assessment and outcome measures, clinicians are increasingly faced with the pragmatic need to objectively document not only the clinical diagnoses they assign but also the methods by which they arrived at these diagnoses. Well-designed structured interviews with a clear recording format provide a logical method for achieving this goal. In summary, structured interviews are an efficient way to provide increased reliability in the diagnostic assessment process.

Advantages of semistructured interviews.   Semistructured interviews, by comparison, are more spontaneous. They provide the clinician with an opportunity to use more clinical judgment in asking questions and in deciding the depth in which each area is to be covered (Edelbrock and Costello 1984). Semistructured interviews have several other advantages over more structured instruments. Because they require an experienced clinician for administration, they can often elicit more precise information about symptom severity rather than simply documenting the presence or absence of a symptom. The clinician uses clinical judgment in making ratings; therefore, he or she has more flexibility in the wording, phrasing, and timing of questions, which can lead to a more natural flow to the interview. However, the person administering the interview must be experienced in child psychopathology to accurately question and probe. Additionally, semistructured interviews tend to be either significantly more time-consuming or less comprehensive in their review of disorders than structured interviews.

Current patterns of use.   In a recent survey of all articles published on "childhood depression" in a 2-year period, Fristad and colleagues (1997) found that 55 of 133 (41%) studies reported using a structured or semistructured interview. The Schedule for Affective Disorders and Schizophrenia for School-Aged Children (Kiddie-SADS; Puig-Antich and Chambers 1978) was by far the most popular interview used (30/55, 55%). Other interviews used in five or more studies were the Diagnostic Interview Schedule for Children (DISC; Costello et al. 1982; 6/55, 11%); the Diagnostic Interview for Children and Adolescents, DSM-III-R Version (DICA-R-C; Reich and Welner 1988; 5/55, 9%); and the Interview Schedule for Children (ISC; Kovacs 1985; 5/55, 9%). Thus, at least in research settings, use of structured and/or semistructured interviews is quite common.

Chapter 3: Development of the Interview

The development of the ChIPS (Weller et al. 1985), a structured interview, proceeded in six phases: 1) reviewing existing interviews; 2) developing a question pool; 3) establishing the interview format; 4) conducting reliability and validity studies; 5) revising the interview to meet DSM-III-R criteria; and 6) revising it to meet DSM-IV criteria. Additional reliability and validity studies have been conducted since the DSM-III-R and DSM-IV revisions were made. These phases—with the exception of Phase IV, the empirical studies, which are discussed in Chapter 5 of this manual—are described below.

Phase I: Reviewing Existing Interviews

The first developmental phase consisted of surveying the available structured diagnostic interviews for children. At the time this review was done, five interviews were available: the Schedule for Affective Disorders and Schizophrenia for School-Aged Children (Kiddie-SADS; Puig-Antich and Chambers 1978), the Interview Schedule for Children (ISC; Kovacs 1985), the Children's Assessment Schedule (CAS; Hodges et al. 1982), the Diagnostic Interview for Children and Adolescents (DICA; Herjanic and Reich 1982), and the Diagnostic Interview Schedule for Children (DISC; Costello et al. 1982). During this review phase, each interview was separated into its component syndromes, and each question was evaluated for age-appropriate language and adherence to DSM-III criteria. This survey resulted in a pool of several hundred questions tapping more than 40 syndromes. Questions pertaining to the syndromes most often seen in the clinical setting were retained; others (e.g., pertaining to Agoraphobia, Transsexualism) were deleted.

Phase II: Developing a Question Pool

The second phase of development consisted of compiling a pool of questions to be tested. Although some questions from Phase I were modified for use, most questions were newly written by the authors. Attention was paid to the content, type, and quality of questions surveyed in the prior phase. Three factors were emphasized in preparing questions. First, wording was monitored to meet appropriate vocabulary guidelines for children ages 6 to 12 years. Second, sentence length was monitored to ensure that children as young as age 6 years (the lower age limit for the interview) could comprehend the questions. Third, questions were designed to be clear, adequately detailed, and easily understood by children. Of note, a study by Breton and colleagues (1995) suggested that comprehensibility of questions in structured interviews is indeed a significant concern. In that study, less than half of the questions of the Diagnostic Interview Schedule for Children—Version 2.25 (DISC-2.25; Shaffer et al. 1991) were correctly understood by a group of 240 elementary school children ages 9 to 11 years. Likewise, only about one-quarter of the children correctly understood the questions regarding time concepts. Thus, attention paid to word selection, question length, and question comprehensibility is critical in the development of a structured interview. Efforts in this regard are discussed below.

Appropriate word selection.   Questions were designed using words within the vocabulary of children ages 6 to 12 years. Simple, short words with literal connotations were chosen (e.g. "Do you try to have fun, but nothing is fun anymore?" instead of "Did you experience a loss of interest or pleasure?"; American Psychiatric Association 1994). When the possibility of ambiguity existed, alternative wordings and clarifications were supplied (e.g., for the question "Do you worry a lot about something bad happening to your parents?" the explanation "like getting sick, being hurt, or dying" is also provided). This material serves two purposes. First, it may be used by the interviewer to help clarify questions if the child does not appear to understand the original question. For example, the Conduct Disorder section includes the question "Have you skipped school [played hooky] several times or more?" If a child does not understand the question, information is provided for the interviewer to further clarify the question by using the alternate wording "Have you *played hooky* several times or more?" The second purpose served by providing alternative wording is that such clarifications may be used by the interviewer to help decide whether the child's response should be counted as an affirmative or negative response. For example, another Conduct Disorder section question is "Have you ever damaged any property (such as breaking windows, scratching up a car, slashing tires or seats on buses)?" Children may answer in the affirmative to a general question about damaging property for a wide variety of offenses they have committed. The clarification statement "such as breaking windows, scratching up a car, slashing tires or seats on buses" should decrease the likelihood of a false-positive response.

Question length.   Question length was the second variable addressed while constructing questions. Harris and Liebert (1987) have reported that young children understand short questions more easily than longer ones. Breton et al. (1995) demonstrated in their study that children are significantly more likely to understand shorter (i.e., 1 to 9 words) as compared with medium-length (i.e., 10 to 19 words) and longer (i.e., 20 or more words) sentences. Questions from the draft ChIPS were brief, averaging 12 words in length. The widely used DICA, considered representative of the highly structured interviews, employs questions averaging 18 words in length.

Comprehensibility.   Proposed questions were read to 23 psychiatrically hospitalized children ages 6 to 11 years, all with IQ levels greater than 70, to determine whether the questions were comprehensible to the children. Based on feedback from this sample, several questions were rewritten and clarified before being included in the DSM-III version of the interview. The result of this process was an interview containing 303 questions distributed across 17 categories.

Phase III: Establishing the Interview Format

The third phase in the development of the ChIPS was to establish the interview format. This involved two important considerations. First, the order in which the individual syndromes were to be covered was established. Second, questions within a given syndrome were ordered along a dimension ranging from global to specific.

Order of syndromes in the ChIPS.   Syndromes were included in the interview schedule in an order that generally reflects their estimated prevalence in the general population (Yule 1981). The most common syndromes are those involving behavior problems (Attention-Deficit/Hyperactivity Disorder, Oppositional Defiant Disorder, Conduct Disorder, and Substance Abuse), and these were included first. Next came the anxiety disorders (Phobias, Separation and Generalized Anxiety Disorders, Obsessive-Compulsive Disorder, and Stress Disorders) and the eating disorders (Anorexia and Bulimia), followed by the mood disorders (Depression/Dysthymia and Mania/Hypomania) and the elimination disorders (Enuresis and Encopresis). Schizophrenia/Psychosis appears as the last of the DSM-IV disorders.

In addition to the clinical syndromes assessed by the ChIPS, a Psychosocial Stressors section was added to screen for child abuse/neglect and other stressors. This was included to help obtain a more complete perspective, because review of these areas is considered to be important in the psychological assessment of the child (Achenbach 1982; Hetherington and Martin 1979). This section follows a modified branching format, such that almost every question in the two subcategories of Child Abuse/Neglect and Other Stressors should be asked routinely. These questions request specific information concerning potentially stressful and sensitive issues. They are included last in the interview because rapport should be well established by then, and the child should be accustomed to the question-and-answer format. These factors should help the child feel more comfortable in dealing with potentially embarrassing or difficult-to-answer questions.

Order of questions within syndromes.   The order of questions within each syndrome was based on a decision to begin with common and/or less threatening symptoms. The first questions in each syndrome are "cardinal" questions, designed to assess the presence or absence of a common or very characteristic symptom of the syndrome. Questions are ordered as listed in the DSM-IV. Those questions concerning symptoms that either have a low incidence of occurrence or are more threatening are asked only after the probable existence of the disorder has been established.

Summary.   These procedural features help make the ChIPS efficient in its administration. The branching format aids in this endeavor. The ChIPS interview progresses in a manner such that the less threatening topic areas are broached at the beginning of the interview and are used to establish rapport. The interview then progresses toward more threatening topic areas. This design facilitates the continued development and maintenance of rapport.

Phase IV: Conducting Reliability and Validity Studies

The research studies conducted to establish the reliability and validity of the ChIPS are discussed in Chapter 5.

Phases V and VI: Revising the Interview to Meet DSM-III-R and DSM-IV Criteria

Since the development of the ChIPS, it has been revised to meet DSM-III-R and DSM-IV criteria. The first revision was the most extensive, because the change in criteria from DSM-III to DSM-III-R was more pronounced than that from DSM-III-R to DSM-IV. This first change involved rewriting questions to correspond with DSM-III-R revisions. Also, questions within each syndrome were reordered to align with the new order of symptoms in DSM-III-R, based on their frequency of occurrence in field trials.

DSM-IV revisions were conducted in the same way. Because of the addition, deletion, and expansion of syndromes (e.g., Overanxious Disorder is now part of Generalized Anxiety Disorder, Acute Stress Disorder has been added, Posttraumatic Stress Disorder has been expanded), corresponding changes were made in the interview. Old questions were kept whenever possible and realigned to fit the new disorders. New questions were written as needed, taking into consideration vocabulary, question length, and comprehensibility.

ChIPS— Parent Version (P-ChIPS)

A parent version of the ChIPS (P-ChIPS) was developed at the same time that the DSM-III-R revisions were being made. This interview is based strictly on the ChIPS and essentially consists of the same interview text altered from second to third person (e.g., "Have you ever" is changed to "Has your child ever"). All questions have a one-to-one correspondence between the ChIPS and the P-ChIPS. This was done to ensure that parents and children are asked similar questions, thereby decreasing potential variability when comparing child and parent reports.

Chapter 4: Administration and Scoring

The ChIPS is designed to be administered face to face. Both the interview and the scoring form are used when assessing a child with the ChIPS. The interview is designed to be administered either by an experienced clinician or by a trained test administrator. The interviewer should not conduct this interview without using both the interview and the scoring form. The interviewer should not try to remember responses and write them down later. There is ample space on the scoring form to record the child's responses. Deviation from this protocol is a departure from the format used in the reliability and validity studies that were conducted on this instrument.

These instructions are meant for individuals who are already familiar with the ChIPS interview and scoring form. The reader should refer to the interview and scoring form as needed while reading this chapter.

In the following sections, the child interview (ChIPS) is used as the example. Administration of the adult interview (P-ChIPS) is to be conducted in the same manner, unless specifically noted.

General Administration Guidelines

Opening Phase

The interviewer should spend several minutes getting to know the child before the diagnostic portion of the interview begins. This is essential for several reasons. First, this preliminary period allows the interviewer to establish rapport, ensuring that the child is comfortable enough with the interviewer to share information. Second, the interviewer will be able to determine whether the child is sufficiently capable, cognitively and emotionally, of completing the interview. Third, the preliminary questions elicit standardized information regarding the child's perception of the reason for referral; his or her overall functioning at home, at school, and with peers; and his or her past treatment history, including use of psychotropic medication.

The interviewer should complete the top section of the scoring form's profile sheet. Information to be recorded includes the child's name and/or identification number, birthdate, age, race, and sex. The interviewer should also include his or her own name and circle the setting in which the interview is being administered (in the case of a parent interview, this should be the setting in which the child is being seen). (For the parent interview, a space is provided on the P-ChIPS profile sheet to record the name of the parent or other informant and his or her relationship to the child.) Also to be recorded is the date and time of administration. The interviewer should record the time the interview begins and the time it ends. If the interview is conducted with breaks, that should be noted as well, so that the total interview time is clear.

The interviewer begins by asking the child whether he or she is having any problems and, if so, what kind. The child's response is recorded verbatim. The interviewer follows with specific questions about the child's home, school, peers, and work (where applicable). The child's responses to all of these questions are recorded verbatim as well. These questions serve two purposes: first, they offer a nonthreatening context in which the interviewer and the child can become acquainted; and second, they provide the interviewer with pertinent information to use later in the interview (such as who the child's primary caretaker is). The medication question provides useful information to the interviewer and the interpreting clinician regarding the child's current treatment.

During this introductory phase, the interviewer should assess the child's cognitive and emotional state. The interview should not be conducted with children who are extremely agitated, mute, stuporous, disoriented, tired, or obviously uncooperative. Because persons with low IQ (e.g., 70 or less) were not included in the reliability and validity studies, responses from such individuals are suspect. In such cases, a parent might be interviewed instead. If the parent's IQ is believed to be below 70, the interview should be administered and interpreted with great caution.

Some children will not be able to remain seated throughout the entire interview. In such cases, the interviewer can allow the child to get up and move about the room, as long as the child's attention remains focused on the questions being asked. If the child is unable to remain focused, a break in the interview is in order. Although a break may occur at any time, it is preferable for it to occur between disorders. The break may be brief (5 to 10 minutes), or the interviewer may choose to resume on the following day. The interviewer should not allow too much time to pass between parts of an interview, however, because the child's condition may improve or deteriorate, thus affecting interpretation of the interview results.

Syndrome Review

Order of presentation. The diagnostic portion of the interview begins with Attention-Deficit/Hyperactivity Disorder and proceeds systematically through the list of 20 disorders listed in the interview booklet.

Questions are asked in the order that they appear in the interview. Answers are recorded and scored on the scoring form *while the interview is in progress*. Scoring criteria for each disorder are presented both in the interview and on the scoring form.

The cardinal questions for each disorder are always asked, regardless of the child's presenting problem. If the child meets the indicated requirements, more questions about the disorder are asked. If child meets full criteria for the disorder, the Duration and Impairment questions are also asked. If the child does not meet the indicated requirements, the interviewer proceeds to the next section of the interview. The exception to this procedure would be if the child (for some reason) did not meet criteria for a disorder (such as depression) but the interviewer believes (e.g., by observation, because it was stated as the child's presenting problem, or because the child is medicated with a known antidepressant) that there is a strong likelihood that the child has the disorder. In such a case, the interviewer may choose to ask further questions in that section and may even return to and reask the cardinal questions with further clarification based on the child's responses.

Wording and use of examples. Questions in the ChIPS are read to the child. Minor changes in wording are allowed, as long as the essential features of the question are clear. The primary goal is to ensure that the child fully understands the intent of the questions. Toward this end, alternative wordings are provided in brackets for some questions.

When a child does not fully understand the meaning of a question, concrete examples may be useful. Such examples are provided in the interview in parentheses. The interviewer can also use his or her own words to explain the question in an appropriate manner. For example, the child may not understand the meaning of the first question in Section B of Obsessive-Compulsive Disorder: "Do you have bothersome ideas or thoughts that keep coming back into your mind over and over again?" The interviewer can clarify *bothersome* by giving examples such as "thinking your hands have germs on them, or that you will harm someone, or that things have to be perfectly even." If the child has indicated an obsession or compulsion as the presenting problem, the interviewer could use that example.

It is important that the child understand the meaning of the cardinal question, because a falsely negative reply would result in incorrectly skipping a section. Conversely, a false-positive response would result in asking unnecessary questions.

Response elaboration. Another way to ensure comprehension is to ask for an example when an affirmative response to a question is given. In some parts of the interview (such as the Obsessive-Compulsive Disorder question above), querying for an example is required. The interviewer can request such an example elsewhere in the interview as needed to verify the child's level of understanding. This may be especially important when dealing with younger children. However, the interviewer should not undertake this with every question, as it could make the interview too cumbersome and tedious. A child whose answers appear to need this much verification may not be an appropriate interview candidate.

Modification of a question. When a child has described a symptom or a problem in the introductory questions or while elaborating on a response to a prior question, the interviewer can use this information by changing the wording of any item pertaining to that symptom. *However, the interviewer should not omit questions that touch on experiences that the child has already described.* Instead, the interviewer should ask the question to reaffirm the child's response. The interviewer may provide further clarification or remind the child of his or her prior response to facilitate questioning. For example, a child may tell the interviewer that he is there because he stole some items from a store and got caught. The ChIPS Conduct Disorder questions may be modified or introduced accordingly:

> "I believe you said you are here because you stole some things and got caught?" Allow child to confirm, then continue with the second half of Question 1 (i.e., "How often?"). If, for example, child's reply is "No, I broke into a car and stole some tapes," the interviewer could rephrase Question 3 to say "and you mentioned that you broke into a car and stole some tapes?" (and allow the child to confirm this again).

Usually a change in verb tense and a brief introductory phrase such as "you said" or "you mentioned" are the only modifications needed to let the child know that you listened to and remembered something previously mentioned.

Duration and Impairment questions may more frequently require some type of modification. The answers to these questions may be obtained from the child's comments during the interview, without further prompting from the interviewer. For example, if a child states that she became depressed in third grade, the interviewer could record this without asking the child when she first had problems with depression. Repeatedly asking questions that the child has already answered may cause the child to become irritated with the interviewer, lose interest in the interview, or otherwise invalidate the process. Similarly, when asking Duration questions, it may become clear that the child's sense of time is not sufficiently developed to allow him or her to answer them. In such cases, Duration questions may need to be discontinued to prevent the child from building up resentment.

Effective use of the branching format. Each section of the ChIPS contains break points that allow the interviewer to skip to the next disorder if certain criteria have not been met. In the majority of cases, the interviewer will have no problem determining whether these criteria have been met. For those rare cases in which doubt exists, the interviewer should ask the remaining questions in the series. In doing so, the interviewer is in a position to clarify any uncertainty that may have arisen and will avoid making a false-negative decision.

Duration questions. Duration questions vary slightly from disorder to disorder. However, their main intent is to establish how old the child was when the problem first occurred or began, whether the problem is still going on, and whether the duration of the problem meets the specified criteria (e.g., for Attention-Deficit/Hyperactivity Disorder, onset prior to age 7 years and duration of at least 6 months). Some children may endorse a sufficient number of symptoms to meet diagnostic criteria for a disorder but not meet the requisite duration criteria for that disorder. This can occur for several reasons—the disorder has not persisted for the specified length of time, the child's sense of time is not well enough developed for him or her to accurately report duration, or the child has a faulty or hazy memory about the onset of symptoms. For such children, the box for Diagnosis can be checked while that for Duration is left blank.

Impairment questions. The intent of the Impairment questions is to determine whether children have experienced any interference in their lives as a result of the aforementioned symptoms in a certain disorder. On the P-ChIPS, Impairment questions should elicit the parent's perception of whether the child is in trouble, not the parent's report of the child's perception of whether he or she is in trouble.

Tempo of the Interview

The speed with which an interview is conducted can vary considerably. Most children will adapt quickly to a fairly steady tempo of questions and responses. A few, particularly younger children, may require more time to ensure that they stay focused on the questions asked and do not get into a response set (i.e., just repeating their earlier responses). Some questions may stimulate a verbose reply from the child. In these cases, it is best to listen supportively at first, then interrupt the child in a kind way, returning him or her to the interview process. One way of doing this would be to say, "I think I understand what you are saying; now I'd like to ask you some more questions."

Recording Answers and Scoring

Scoring Form and Profile Sheet

The syndromes are arranged on the scoring form in the same order that they appear in the interview. The letters within brackets refer to the alphabetic subparts of the question (e.g., 1. <a> <b> refers to Part a and Part b of Question 1). When the child responds in the affirmative, the interviewer should mark a slash through the appropriate box. A negative response should be indicated by circling the box. An empty box signifies that the question was not asked. *As a rule, ChIPS questions are written so that an affirmative response is considered a symptom endorsement.* For age-related questions or questions that are open-ended in nature, blank lines are provided on the scoring form to record the child's response(s). Criteria for each disorder are listed on the scoring form. They appear after the last symptom question but before the Duration and Impairment questions. A box is provided in which to record whether symptom criteria have been met, as well as a box to note whether duration requirements (if any) have also been met. After completion of the interview, this information should be transferred to the profile sheet to facilitate review of ChIPS results. Additionally, if a child reported subthreshold symptoms of a disorder, this should be noted on the profile sheet in the column labeled Symptoms. It is important that the Symptoms, Diagnosis, and Duration boxes all be used. Doing so will allow this important information to be conveyed in a concise manner.

Optional Report Form

The optional report form may be used to easily document endorsements made by a child or parent on the ChIPS or P-ChIPS. If this is desired, several steps should be followed upon completion of the interview. First, the child's name and the date of the interview must be recorded on page 3 of the scoring form and on page 1 of the report form. Second, the completed profile sheet can be detached from the scoring form (the sheet is perforated to allow this) and attached to the report form. Finally, positive item endorsements from the scoring form can be indicated by circling the appropriate question numbers on the report form.

Sample Forms

Sample portions of the scoring form, the profile sheet, and the report form are presented in Figures 1, 2, and 3, respectively. These samples are based on an interview with a 13-year-old boy who presented to an outpatient clinic with behavior problems.

Page 3 of the scoring form (Figure 1) indicates that 11 questions were endorsed in the Attention-Deficit/ Hyperactivity Disorder (ADHD) section (questions regarding making careless mistakes, not listening to teachers, not finishing chores, having trouble getting organized, losing supplies, daydreaming, being called forgetful, getting in trouble for running or climbing, talking out of turn, pushing ahead in line, and barging into kids' games). Symptoms were noted to begin at age 3, and most continued to cause significant problems for him at home, with peers, and at school. The Diagnosis and Duration boxes for ADHD should be checked on the profile sheet (i.e., the first page of the scoring form) (Figure 2). For Oppositional Defiant Disorder (ODD), 5 symptoms were endorsed (losing temper, arguing with parents, breaking house rules, "bugging" others, and blaming others for his problems). Symptoms began at age 8 and have remained highly problematic. Thus, the Diagnosis and Duration boxes for ODD should be checked on the profile sheet. For Conduct Disorder (CD), only stealing and lying were endorsed. For this disorder, Duration and Impairment questions were not asked because the child did not meet diagnostic criteria. Therefore, only the Symptoms box for CD on the profile sheet should be checked. The "at-a-glance" symptom summary contained in the completed report form (Figure 3) enables a clinician to quickly identify areas that warrant further scrutiny.

Child's Name: _John Smith_

Date: _4/21/99_

ADHD	ODD	CD
A. Inattention 1. (a) b Always! 2. < > 3. (a) b ditto 4. a b c 5. room's a mess 6. < > 7. 8. (a) b every day! 9. (a) b both B. Hyperactivity–Impulsivity 1. (a) (b) 2. (a) (b) 3. furniture 4. (a) (b) 5. < > 6. a b just got moved 7. < > d/t this 8. a b detention 9. a b c esp. @ baseball practice	1. a b friends tease about 2. a b grounded this 3. a b c d grounded 4. 5. (a) b 6. < > 7. < > 8. < >	1. 2x- yrs ago 2. a b all the time 3. < > 4. < > 5. < > 6. < > 7. (a) (b) 8. (a) (b) 9. < > 10. (a) (b) 11. < > 12. < > 13. < > 14. < > 15. (a) (b)
Criteria If ≥6 in *A only*, then criteria met Inattentive ✓ If ≥6 in *B only*, then criteria met Hyperactive–Impulsive < > If ≥6 in A *and* ≥6 in B, then criteria met Combined < >	**Criteria** If ≥4, then criteria met ODD ✓	**Criteria** If ≥3, then criteria met CD < >
Duration Mom says I was "a maniac" in 1. ___3___ (years old) pre 2. ✓ _13_ (years old) school 3. ✓ _120_ (months) * DUR met for ADHD ✓	**Duration** started getting in more trouble 1. ___8___ (years old) 2. ✓ _13_ (years old) 3. ✓ _60_ (months) 3rd gr. * DUR met for ODD ✓	**Duration** 1. _____ (years old) 2. < > _____ (years old) 3. < > _____ (months) * DUR met for CD < >
Impairment 1. ✓ home 2. ✓ school 3. ✓ peers Parents - always yelling abt homework Tchr - "gets on my case" Baseball - "a bust"	**Impairment** 1. ✓ home 2. ✓ school 3. ✓ peers "My pals get annoyed w me" Tchr - "tells me I'm too hot headed" Soccer coach - "said I had 'an attitude' + didn't want me back"	**Impairment** 1. < > home 2. < > school 3. < > peers **Type** Childhood Onset < > Adolescent Onset < > Mild < > Moderate < > Severe < >

Figure 1. Sample page of scoring form for interview with 13-year-old boy presenting to outpatient clinic with behavior problems.

Child's Number: _906-43-7941_ Date: _4/21/99_

Child's Name: _John Smith_ Time Started: _1:05 pm_

Date of Birth: _10/15/85_ Age: _13 1/2_ Time Ended: _1:40 pm_

Race: _Caucasian_ Sex: _M_ Interviewer: _Mary Jones, M.A._

Setting (circle one): Inpatient, (Outpatient,) School, Other Research Setting: _____

	Disorder	Symptoms	Diagnosis	Duration	Clinician's Diagnosis
ADHD	Attention-Deficit/Hyperactivity Disorder	<>	✓	✓	Axis I
	Type: (Inattentive,) Hyperactive–Impulsive, Combined				ADHD
					ODD
ODD	Oppositional Defiant Disorder	<>	✓	✓	
CD	Conduct Disorder	✓	<>	<>	
	Onset: Childhood, Adolescent				
	Severity: Mild, Moderate, Severe				
SUBAB	Substance Abuse	<>	<>	<>	
	Substance(s): _____				
PHO	Specific Phobia	<>	<>	<>	Axis II
	Type: _____				∅
SOCPHO	Social Phobia	<>	<>	<>	
SEPANX	Separation Anxiety Disorder	<>	<>	<>	Axis III
GENANX	General Anxiety Disorder	<>	<>	<>	∅
OCD	Obsessive-Compulsive Disorder	<>	<>	<>	
PTSD	Posttraumatic Stress Disorder	<>	<>	<>	Axis IV
	Type: Acute, Chronic				recent
	Onset: Regular, Delayed				Separation
ASD	Acute Stress Disorder	<>	<>	<>	
ANO	Anorexia	<>	<>	<>	Axis V
BUL	Bulimia	<>	<>	<>	current: 60
DEP	Major Depressive Disorder	<>	<>	<>	past year: 75
DYS	Dysthymic Disorder	<>	<>	<>	
MAN	Mania	<>	<>	<>	
HYPOMAN	Hypomania	<>	<>	<>	
ENU	Enuresis	<>	<>	<>	
	Type: Nocturnal, Diurnal, Both				
ENC	Encopresis	<>	<>	<>	
SCZ	Schizophrenia	<>	<>	<>	
PSY	Psychosis	<>	<>	<>	

Psychosocial Stressors: _parents separated 8 mos ago_

Other Stressors: _∅_

Behavioral Observations

Appearance: _neatly groomed, casually dressed_ Affect: _mildly nervous initially— then settled into interview_

Effort: _adequate_ Level of Activity: _fidgeted_

Unusual Behaviors: _∅_

Figure 2. Sample profile sheet for interview with 13-year-old boy presenting to outpatient clinic with behavior problems.

Child's Name: _John Smith_ Date: _4_ / _21_ / _99_

Interviewer: _Mary Jones, M.A._

Attention-Deficit/Hyperactivity Disorder

A: Inattention

1. a. pays no attention to details
   (b) makes careless mistakes on schoolwork *always*
2. can't keep mind on what he/she is doing
3. a. has trouble listening to parent
   (b) has trouble listening to teacher *always*
(4) has trouble finishing things
(5) has trouble organizing self *esp. bedroom*
6. avoids schoolwork
(7) loses school supplies
8. a. is easily distracted
   (b) teacher reports inattention/daydreaming *every day!*
9. a. is forgetful
   (b) teacher reports forgetfulness *+ parents = parents*

B: Hyperactivity–Impulsivity

1. a. is often told to sit still
   b. is constantly moving hands/feet
2. a. has trouble staying in seat
   b. gets in trouble for getting out of chair
(3) gets in trouble for running/climbing *furniture*
4. a. is too loud when playing
   b. has difficulty playing quietly
5. teacher reports is always "on the go"
6. (a) talks out of turn at school *moved in class*
   b. talks too much at home *b/c of this*
7. blurts out answers to questions
8. (a) pushes ahead in line *one detention*
   b. can't wait for his/her turn in games
9. (a) barges in on other kids' games *baseball practice*
   b. pushes into others' groups
   c. interrupts busy people

Oppositional Defiant Disorder

1. (a) loses temper when things don't go his/her way
   b. has frequent temper tantrums *causes problems/ teasing*
rounded [2. (a) talks back/argues with parents
   b. talks back/argues with teachers
[3. (a) breaks rules at home
   b. breaks rules at school
   c. refuses to follow teachers' directions
   d. disobeys direct orders
(4) purposely "bugs" other people
(5) blames others for his/her own mistakes
6. is easily angered by others
7. is angry a lot of the time
8. gets even when angered

Conduct Disorder

(1) has stolen >1 time *2x - years ago*
2. (a) lies to get out of doing things *all the time*
   b. "cons" people
3. has broken into a car or building to steal
4. has skipped school >3 times
5. breaks curfew >1 time per month
6. has run away/stayed out all night >1 time *or* did not return for a long time
7. a. is a bully
   b. threatens other people
8. a. is avoided because he/she starts fights
   b. gets in trouble for fighting
9. has used a weapon in a fight >1 time
10. a. has hurt someone badly in a fight
    b. has hurt someone for no reason
11. has taken things from people by force
12. has damaged property
13. has set something on fire (>1 time *or* caused extensive damage)
14. has hurt or killed an animal for fun
15. a. has forcefully performed sexual activity on another
    b. has forced someone to perform sexual activity on him-/herself

Substance Abuse

1. a. has smoked cigarettes ≥2 times _____
   b. has smoked pot ≥2 times _____
   c. has smoked other drugs ≥2 times _____
2. has used alcohol _____
3. has used other drugs _____
4. has sniffed a substance ≥2 times _____

Figure 3. Sample page of report form for interview with 13-year-old boy presenting to outpatient clinic with behavior problems.

Chapter 5: Psychometric Properties: Studies of Reliability and Validity

Research studies have been conducted over a 12-year period to examine the reliability and validity of the ChIPS. Children in these studies were in nonoverlapping groups unless clearly stated otherwise. Interviews for the studies were conducted by interviewers with training similar to that outlined in this manual. They included psychology graduate students, advanced undergraduate psychology honors students, medical students, and other medical personnel (e.g., child psychiatrists, staff nurses). Informed consent was obtained from the parents of all participants, assent was obtained from all participants, and measures were taken to ensure confidentiality.

Reliability

Each interviewer was trained according to the methods outlined in this manual. At the conclusion of the training period and prior to the beginning of the study, interrater reliability was assessed. A minimum interrater reliability coefficient of .90 was required before interviewers were permitted to participate in actual data collection. Calculations were performed by comparing the scoring of videotaped interviews with the original interviewers' scoring. Once data collection began, the trainer observed and scored each interview that a trainee conducted with an actual research participant to ensure 90% interrater reliability for individual questions and the diagnosis. When resources permitted, interviewers conducted random checks of each other's work to provide additional quality assurance. In no instance did a researcher fall below this 90% cutoff rate.

Validity

A series of five studies provided validity data for the ChIPS (Fristad et al. 1998a, 1998b, 1998c; Teare et al. 1998a, 1998b). Four of these studies examined the child version and one study examined the parent version (P-ChIPS) of the instrument. The methodology and results of these studies are summarized below.

Study I: Development and Criterion Validity of the ChIPS

In this initial study (Teare et al. 1998a), we administered both the original DSM-III version of the ChIPS and the DSM-III version of the Diagnostic Interview for Children and Adolescents (DICA; Herjanic and Reich 1982) to 42 children ages 6 to 12 years hospitalized in a children's inpatient unit using a counterbalanced Latin Square design (i.e., each instrument was administered first half of the time, each interviewer administered equal numbers of the two instruments, and each interviewer went first half of the time). Most children were administered the ChIPS and the DICA within a 48-hour interval; all were tested within a 1-week interval. A standard kappa coefficient or a rare kappa coefficient and percentage agreement were used to calculate the level of agreement regarding the presence or absence of 15 syndromes/diagnoses as assessed by the two instruments (Table 1). Agreement between the two instruments was significant ($P < .05$) for 13 of the 14 diagnoses for which either type of kappa coefficient could be calculated; agreement was 98% for the remaining diagnosis, Bulimia, which had a nonsignificant kappa. A kappa coefficient could not be calculated for Anorexia because of 100% agreement on its absence. ChIPS and DICA results were also compared with a psychiatrist's diagnosis to establish criterion validity. Sensitivity was 80% for the ChIPS and 61% for the DICA. Specificity was 78% for the ChIPS and 87% for the DICA. In 72% of cases, all three sources agreed (Table 2). Disagreements were most commonly due to one or both of the structured interviews producing a diagnosis not made by the psychiatrist because of hierarchical decision making (i.e., the clinician would diagnose only Conduct Disorder, whereas the ChIPS produced endorsements for Conduct Disorder and Oppositional Defiant Disorder; see comment to Case Report 1 in Chapter 6 of this manual) or because of the secondary diagnosis's lesser importance clinically (e.g., Phobia).

Study II: Reliability and Validity of the DSM-III-R ChIPS

For the second study (Teare et al. 1998b), 71 psychiatric inpatients and outpatients ages 6 to 13 years were recruited from two midwestern cities. They were administered the DSM-III-R–revised ChIPS and the DSM-III-R–revised Diagnostic Interview for Children and Adolescents (DICA-R-C; Reich and Welner 1988). Clinicians' diagnoses were recorded for 26 of the patients. Comparisons between diagnostic sources were made by using percentage agreement and either a standard or a rare kappa coefficient (Table 3). High levels of agreement were found between the two interviews on all 14 syndromes analyzed ($P < .05$). Next, ChIPS results were compared with the clinician diagnoses. Sensitivity and specificity were calculated for each diagnosis (Table 4). Sensitivity ranged from 0% (for Anorexia and Mania) to 100% (for Overanxious Disorder) and averaged 48%. Specificity ranged from 57% (for Attention-Deficit Hyperactivity Disorder) to 100% (for Anorexia and Bulimia) and averaged 86%. When all three diagnostic sources were compared, ChIPS results, DICA-R-C results, and clinician diagnoses agreed 68% of the time. When there was disagreement among the three sources regarding a syndrome's presence, ChIPS–clinician agreement was 47.5%, while DICA-R-C–clinician agreement was 37.5%. For 15% of clinician diagnoses, the diagnosis was made only by the clinician and not by either interview. Total administration times was significantly less for the ChIPS than for the DICA-R-C (M ± SD [minutes]: 42.5 ± 14.9 vs. 65.2 ± 21.0, $t = 6.55$, $df = 104$, $P < .0001$). This finding was true for both inpatients (M ± SD: 46.0 ± 15.9 vs. 68.0 ± 20.5, $t = 5.00$, $df = 68$, $P < .0001$) and outpatients (M ± SD: 35.7 ± 9.7 vs. 59.7 ± 19.1, $t = 4.71$, $df = 34$, $P < .0001$). On the average, administration time was 23 minutes less for the ChIPS than for the DICA-R-C.

Study III: Reliability and Validity of the P-ChIPS

In the third study (Fristad et al. 1998a), the parent versions of the ChIPS (P-ChIPS) and the DICA-R-C (DICA-R-P) were administered to the parents of a subsample of 36 participants from Study II. Additionally, P-ChIPS results were compared with clinician diagnoses for 21 of the children using either a standard or a rare kappa coefficient and percentage agreement. Results indicated 1) moderate levels of agreement between the parent and child versions of the instrument, consistent with other reports of parent–child concordance on structured interviews in the literature (Table 5); and 2) moderate levels of agreement between the parent interview and clinician diagnoses, again consistent with other reports of parent–clinician concordance in the literature (Table 6) (refer to Fristad et al. 1998a for a thorough review of these results). Sensitivity averaged 87% across diagnostic categories; specificity averaged 76%. These findings suggest that the P-ChIPS has adequate validity for use in clinical settings.

Study IV: Children's Interview for Psychiatric Syndromes (ChIPS)—Revised Psychometrics for DSM-IV

In the fourth study (Fristad et al. 1998b), 47 psychiatric inpatients ages 6 to 12 years ($n = 23$) and 13 to 18 years ($n = 24$) were administered the DSM-IV–revised ChIPS and 40 participants were administered the DICA-R-C. In addition, discharge diagnoses were recorded for all participants. Standard kappas, low-base-rate kappas, and percentage agreement were used to assess diagnostic agreement between the two instruments for 18 disorders. High levels of agreement were found between ChIPS and DICA-R-C results (Table 7) as well as between ChIPS results and discharge diagnoses (Table 8). Of the 16 ChIPS–DICA-R-C kappas calculated, 14 were significant ($P < .05$); 2 disorders had 98% agreement but nonsignificant kappa coefficients ($\kappa_x = .494$, $P < .157$). Kappa coefficients could not be calculated for the remaining 2 disorders (Anorexia, Bulimia) because of 100% agreement on their absence. When ChIPS results were compared with discharge diagnoses, sensitivity for each disorder averaged 70% while specificity averaged 84% (see Table 8). When the three sources failed to agree, the ChIPS results were somewhat more likely than the DICA-R-C results (27% vs. 22%) to agree with the discharge diagnoses. Analyses were repeated for children and adolescents (Table 9) and for boys and girls (Table 10). Boys and children had fewer significant ChIPS–DICA-R-C kappa coefficients compared with girls and adolescents; this appeared related to the fewer syndromes they endorsed. ChIPS–clinician agreement was similar for boys and girls as well as for children and adolescents. Administration time was less for the ChIPS than for the DICA-R-C (M ± SD [minutes]: 48.9 ± 11.6 vs. 53.5 ± 15.8, $t = 1.81$, $df = 39$, $P < .08$).

Study V: Children's Interview for Psychiatric Syndromes (ChIPS): Psychometrics in Two Community Samples

In this final study (Fristad et al. 1998c), 40 children ages 6 to 18 years from a community sample ($n = 22$) and from a bereaved sample 1 to 2 years post–parental death ($n = 18$) were interviewed with the ChIPS and the DICA-R-C in a Latin Square design. A consensus panel of child psychopathology experts determined the presence or absence of syndromes/symptoms after reviewing assessment materials not including the ChIPS. Results indicate that the ChIPS' sensitivity is commensurate with epidemiological base rates (17.5% of participants endorsed at least one syndrome). Low-base-rate kappas and percentage agreement were calculated to determine agreement on symptom/syndrome endorsement for 20 disorders (Tables 11 through 14). For syndrome analyses, kappas could not be calculated for more than half of the disorders because of 100% agreement on their absence. For symptom analyses, kappas could not be calculated for 3 of 20 disorders (again, because of 100% agreement on their absence). Of the 17 ChIPS–DICA-R-C symptom kappas calculated, 11 were significant ($P < .04$), 2 had 95% agreement (kappas: $P < .08$), and 4 had 97.5% agreement but nonsignificant kappa coefficients (kappas: $P < .16$). Of the 17 ChIPS–consensus panel symptom kappas, 13 were significant ($P < .04$) and 4 had 97.5% agreement but nonsignificant kappa coefficients (kappas: $P < .16$). In summary, it appears that the validity of the ChIPS in nonclinical samples compares favorably with that of other structured interviews. In addition, the ChIPS required less time to administer than did the DICA-R-C (M ± SD [minutes] 21.3 ± 9.1 vs. 24.3 ± 5.2; $t = 2.76$, $df = 9$, $P < .02$).

Summary

This series of five studies demonstrated the validity of the DSM-III, DSM-III-R–revised, and DSM-IV–revised versions of the ChIPS as well as the validity of the P-ChIPS. Two of the studies examined only psychiatric inpatients, two examined both inpatients and outpatients, and one examined children from two community samples. Three studies focused exclusively on children, whereas two studies examined both children and adolescents. Cumulatively, these studies have demonstrated that 1) the ChIPS provides accurate diagnoses for clinically disturbed populations of children and adolescents; 2) the P-ChIPS is useful in the assessment of childhood psychopathology; 3) the ChIPS is effective in nonclinical settings, such as schools and epidemiological studies (i.e., compared with children from clinical samples, those from nonclinical samples endorse few symptoms and even fewer syndromes); and 4) the ChIPS is brief to administer. Three of these studies compared administration times for the ChIPS and the DICA-R-C. In each case, the ChIPS was significantly quicker to administer. Average administration times were 49 minutes for inpatients, 36 minutes for outpatients, and 21 minutes for community-based children.

Table 1. Agreement on Syndrome Endorsement Between the ChIPS and the DICA: Study I (42 Child Psychiatric Inpatients Ages 6 to 12 Years)

Syndrome	κ^a	$P <$	Agreement (%)	Yes/Yes[b]	No/No[c]
Attention-deficit disorder	.387	.01	69	13	16
Oppositional disorder	.364	.005	74	25	6
Conduct disorder, aggressive	.314	.005	62	13	13
Conduct disorder, nonaggressive	.309	.006	62	11	15
Phobic disorder	.432[a]	.0006	76	0	32
Separation anxiety disorder	.525[a]	.0001	76	3	29
Overanxious disorder	.455[a]	.003	83	0	35
Obsessive-compulsive disorder	.601[a]	.01	93	1	38
Anorexia[d]	—	—	100	0	42
Bulimia	.494[a]	.16	98	0	41
Depressive episode	.474[a]	.0001	64	6	21
Manic episode	.482[a]	.04	93	0	39
Schizophrenia	.731[a]	.006	95	2	38
Enuresis	.731[a]	.0001	88	7	30
Encopresis	.475[a]	.02	90	0	38

Note. ChIPS = Children's Interview for Psychiatric Syndromes. DICA = Diagnostic Interview for Children and Adolescents.

[a]Regular kappa (κ) was used except where rare kappa (Verducci et al. 1988) is indicated with footnote.

[b]Number of cases in which the syndrome was scored as present by both interviews.

[c]Number of cases in which the syndrome was scored as absent by both interviews.

[d]Coefficient could not be computed because of perfect agreement on absence of disorder.

Table 2. Concordance Between ChIPS Results, DICA Results, and Clinician Diagnoses: Study I (42 Child Psychiatric Inpatients Ages 6 to 12 Years)

		Clinician Diagnosis		
		Negative No. (%)	Positive No. (%)	
DICA Negative	ChIPS Negative	420 (67)	10 (1.6)	430 (68.6)
	ChIPS Positive	75 (12)	13 (2)	88 (14)
DICA Positive	ChIPS Negative	26 (4)	2 (0.3)	28 (4.3)
	ChIPS Positive	50 (8)	34 (5)	84 (13)
		571 (91)	59 (8.9)	630 (100)

Note. Analysis yields 630 potential diagnoses (42 patients × 15 disorders). ChIPS = Children's Interview for Psychiatric Syndromes. DICA = Diagnostic Interview for Children and Adolescents.

Table 3. Agreement on Syndrome Endorsement Between the ChIPS and the DICA-R-C: Study II (71 Child Psychiatric Inpatients and Outpatients Ages 6 to 13 Years)

Syndrome	κ^a	$P <$	Agreement (%)	Yes/Yes[b]	No/No[c]
Attention-deficit hyperactivity disorder	.587	.0001	80	21	36
Oppositional defiant disorder	.570	.0001	79	23	33
Conduct disorder	.570[a]	.0001	77	8	47
Phobic disorder[d]	.542[a]	.0001	78	5	49
Separation anxiety disorder	.512	.0001	77	16	39
Overanxious disorder	.526	.0001	79	16	40
Obsessive-compulsive disorder	.585[a]	.0001	80	7	50
Anorexia[e]	—	—	100	0	71
Bulimia	.745[a]	.04	99	1	69
Depressive episode[d]	.284	.008	65	16	29
Dysthymic disorder[d]	.521[a]	.0001	71	8	39
Manic episode	.523[a]	.0001	76	5	49
Enuresis	.665[a]	.0001	87	7	55
Encopresis[d]	.684[a]	.003	96	2	65

Note. ChIPS = Children's Interview for Psychiatric Syndromes. DICA-R-C = DSM-III-R–revised Diagnostic Interview for Children and Adolescents.

[a]Regular kappa (κ) was used except where rare kappa (Verducci et al. 1988) is indicated with footnote.

[b]Number of cases in which the syndrome was scored as present by both interviews.

[c]Number of cases in which the syndrome was scored as absent by both interviews.

[d]Several syndromes had missing data (phobia, $n = 69$; depression, $n = 69$; dysthymia, $n = 66$; encopresis, $n = 70$).

[e]Coefficient could not be computed because of perfect agreement on absence of disorder.

Table 4. Concordance, Sensitivity, and Specificity for ChIPS Results Versus Clinician Diagnoses: Study II (26 Child Psychiatric Inpatients and Outpatients Ages 6 to 13 Years)

Syndrome	κ^a	$P <$	Agreement (%)	Sensitivity[b] (%)	Specificity[c] (%)
Attention-deficit hyperactivity disorder	−.182	NS	42	25	57
Oppositional defiant disorder	−.013	NS	54	30	69
Conduct disorder	.641	.0004	85	67	94
Phobic disorder	.490[a]	.16	96	—[d]	96
Separation anxiety disorder	.590[a]	.0001	77	80	76
Overanxious disorder	.604[a]	.0004	81	100	78
Obsessive-compulsive disorder	.548[a]	.006	85	50	88
Anorexia	—[d]	—	100	—[d]	100
Bulimia	—[d]	—	100	—[d]	100
Depressive episode	.225	.12	65	40	81
Dysthymic disorder	.458[a]	.02	85	—[d]	85
Manic episode	.435[a]	.006	77	0	87
Enuresis	.536[a]	.0007	77	33	90
Encopresis	.717[a]	.006	92	50	100

Note. ChIPS = Children's Interview for Psychiatric Syndromes.

[a]Regular kappa (κ) was used except where rare kappa (Verducci et al. 1988) is indicated with footnote.

[b]Number of true positive ChIPS endorsements divided by total number of positive clinician endorsements.

[c]Number of true negative ChIPS endorsements divided by total number of negative clinician endorsements.

[d]Coefficient could not be computed because of no endorsement of the disorder by the clinician.

Table 5. Parent–Child Agreement on Syndrome Endorsement Between the P-ChIPS and the ChIPS: Study III (36 Child Psychiatric Inpatients and Outpatients Ages 6 to 13 Years)

Syndrome	κ[a]	$P <$	Agreement (%)	Yes/Yes[b]	No/No[c]
Attention-deficit hyperactivity disorder	.122	NS	50	11	7
Oppositional defiant disorder	.198	.07	56	11	9
Conduct disorder	.432	.003	72	9	17
Phobic disorder	.400[a]	.0003	67	0	24
Separation anxiety disorder	.492[a]	.00001	67	5	19
Overanxious disorder	.160	NS	61	6	16
Obsessive-compulsive disorder[d]	.498[a]	.0001	74	2	24
Anorexia[e]	—	—	100	0	36
Bulimia[e]	—	—	100	0	36
Depressive episode	.452[a]	.00001	61	6	16
Dysthymic disorder	.440[a]	.00001	61	4	18
Manic episode	.449[a]	.0001	67	2	22
Hypomanic episode	.449[a]	.0001	67	2	22
Psychosis	.438[a]	.002	78	0	28
Enuresis	.549[a]	.0001	78	3	25
Encopresis[d]	.596[a]	.01	91	1	31

Note. P-ChIPS = Children's Interview for Psychiatric Syndromes—Parent Version. ChIPS = Children's Interview for Psychiatric Syndromes.

[a]Regular kappa (κ) was used except where rare kappa (Verducci et al. 1988) is indicated with footnote.

[b]Number of cases in which the syndrome was scored as present by both interviews.

[c]Number of cases in which the syndrome was scored as absent by both interviews.

[d]Data for syndrome were missing for some interviews ($n = 35$).

[e]Coefficient could not be computed because of perfect agreement on absence of disorder.

Table 6. Concordance, Sensitivity, and Specificity for P-ChIPS Results Versus Clinician Diagnoses: Study III (21 Child Psychiatric Inpatients and Outpatients Ages 6 to 13 Years)

Syndrome	κ^a	$P <$	Agreement (%)	Sensitivity[b] (%)	Specificity[c] (%)
Attention-deficit hyperactivity disorder	.486	.004	76	100	44
Oppositional defiant disorder	.055	NS	48	75	31
Conduct disorder	.710	.0003	86	100	79
Phobic disorder	.447[a]	.02	81	—[d]	81
Separation anxiety disorder	.710[a]	.0005	86	80	88
Overanxious disorder	.473[a]	.0009	67	67	67
Obsessive-compulsive disorder[d]	.811[a]	.01	95	100	95
Anorexia	—[e]	—	100	—[e]	100
Bulimia	—[e]	—	100	—[e]	100
Depressive episode	.028	NS	52	100	53
Dysthymic disorder	.344[a]	.002	52	—[e]	52
Manic episode	.473[a]	.0009	67	100	63
Hypomanic episode	.475[a]	.07	90	—[e]	90
Psychosis	.462[a]	.04	86	—[e]	86
Enuresis	.673	.0007	86	83	87
Encopresis[d]	.708[a]	.005	90	67	94

Note. P-ChIPS = Children's Interview for Psychiatric Syndromes—Parent Version.

[a]Regular kappa (κ) was used except where rare kappa (Verducci et al. 1988) is indicated with footnote.

[b]Number of true positive ChIPS endorsements divided by total number of positive clinician endorsements.

[c]Number of true negative ChIPS endorsements divided by total number of negative clinician endorsements.

[d]Data for syndrome were missing for some interviews ($n = 35$).

[e]Coefficient could not be computed because of perfect agreement on absence of disorder.

Table 7. Agreement on Syndrome Endorsement Between the ChIPS and the DICA-R-C: Study IV (40 Child and Adolescent Psychiatric Inpatients Ages 6 to 18 Years)

Syndrome	κ^a	$P <$	Agreement (%)	Yes/Yes[b]	No/No[c]
Attention-deficit/hyperactivity disorder	.451	.002	78	7	24
Oppositional defiant disorder	.506	.001	75	17	13
Conduct disorder	.750	.001	88	19	16
Substance abuse	.649[a]	.02	95	1	37
Simple phobia	.638[a]	.001	88	3	32
Social phobia	.718[a]	.001	93	3	34
Separation anxiety disorder	.578[a]	.001	78	5	26
Generalized anxiety disorder	.549[a]	.001	83	2	31
Obsessive-compulsive disorder	.494[a]	.157	98	0	39
Posttraumatic stress disorder	.752[a]	.001	93	4	33
Anorexia	—[d]	—	100	0	40
Bulimia	—[d]	—	100	0	40
Major depressive disorder	.604	.001	80	16	16
Dysthymic disorder	.781	.001	90	12	24
Manic episode	.474[a]	.021	90	0	36
Enuresis	.887[a]	.001	98	4	35
Encopresis	.492[a]	.157	98	0	39
Psychosis	.781	.001	90	12	24

Note. ChIPS = Children's Interview for Psychiatric Syndromes. DICA-R-C = DSM-III-R–revised Diagnostic Interview for Children and Adolescents.

[a]Low-base-rate kappa (κ_x) was used when there was less than 25% endorsement on both the ChIPS and the DICA-R-C, as indicated with footnote.

[b]Number of cases in which the syndrome was scored as present by both interviews.

[c]Number of cases in which the syndrome was scored as absent by both interviews.

[d]Kappa coefficients could not be determined for these syndromes because of 100% agreement on their absence.

Table 8. Concordance, Sensitivity, and Specificity for ChIPS Results Versus Clinician Diagnoses: Study IV (47 Child and Adolescent Psychiatric Inpatients Ages 6 to 18 Years)

Syndrome	κ^{a}	$P <$	Agreement (%)	Sensitivity[b] (%)	Specificity[c] (%)
Attention-deficit/hyperactivity disorder	.363	.01	74	50	85
Oppositional defiant disorder	.306 [a]	.00001	43	67	39
Conduct disorder	.421	.003	70	84	61
Substance abuse	.676[a]	.003	94	67	95
Simple phobia	.460 [a]	.003	85	—[d]	74
Social phobia	.478[a]	.02	91	—[d]	91
Separation anxiety disorder	.678[a]	.0001	89	100	88
Generalized anxiety disorder	.460[a]	.003	85	—[d]	85
Obsessive-compulsive disorder	.495[a]	.16	98	—[d]	98
Posttraumatic stress disorder	.618[a]	.0002	87	100	86
Anorexia	—[e]	—	100	—	100
Bulimia	—[e]	—	100	—	100
Major depressive disorder	.394	.003	89	88	57
Dysthymic disorder	.482[a]	.00001	66	60	68
Manic episode	.781[a]	.002	96	80	100
Enuresis	.466 [a]	.006	87	0	89
Encopresis	—[e]	—	100	—	100
Psychosis	.511	.0008	79	71	82

Note.   ChIPS = Children's Interview for Psychiatric Syndromes.

[a]Regular kappa (κ) was used except where rare kappa (Verducci et al. 1988) is indicated with footnote. Rare kappas were used whenever there was less than 25% endorsement both by the clinician and on the ChIPS.

[b]Number of true positive ChIPS endorsements divided by total number of positive clinician endorsements.

[c]Number of true negative ChIPS endorsements divided by total number of negative clinician endorsements.

[d]Coefficient could not be computed because of no endorsement of the disorder by the clinician.

[e]Coefficient could not be computed because of no endorsement of the disorder by the clinician or on the ChIPS.

Table 9. Agreement on Syndrome Endorsement Between the ChIPS and the DICA-R-C: Study IV (18 Female and 22 Male Psychiatric Inpatients Ages 6 to 18 Years)

Syndrome	Girls					Boys				
	κ^a	P <	Agreement (%)	Yes/Yes[b]	No/No[c]	κ^a	P <	Agreement (%)	Yes/Yes[b]	No/No[c]
Attention-deficit/hyperactivity disorder	.520[a]	.006	78	1	13	.522	.007	77	6	11
Oppositional defiant disorder	.259	.098	89	4	12	.697	.001	86	15	4
Conduct disorder	.769[a]	.001	61	4	7	.637	.001	86	13	6
Substance abuse	.727[a]	.04	94	1	16	.488[a]	.156	95	0	21
Simple phobia	.700[a]	.006	89	2	14	.577[a]	.010	86	1	18
Social phobia	.743[a]	.002	89	3	13	.488[a]	.156	95	0	21
Separation anxiety disorder	.628[a]	.003	83	2	13	.542[a]	.001	73	3	13
Generalized anxiety disorder	.524[a]	.002	72	2	11	.476[a]	.075	91	0	20
Obsessive-compulsive disorder	.486[a]	.156	94	0	17	—[d]	—	100	0	22
Posttraumatic stress disorder	.769[a]	.001	89	4	12	.488[a]	.156	95	0	21
Anorexia	—[d]	—	100	0	18	—[d]	—	100	0	22
Bulimia	—[d]	—	100	0	18	—[d]	—	100	0	22
Major depressive disorder	.649	.002	83	10	5	.522	.007	77	6	11
Dysthymic disorder	.775	.001	89	7	9	.804[a]	.001	91	5	15
Manic episode	.455[a]	.038	83	0	15	.488[a]	.156	95	0	21
Enuresis	.727[a]	.037	94	1	16	1.00[a]	.073	100	3	19
Encopresis	.486[a]	.156	94	0	17	—[d]	—	100	0	22
Psychosis	.886	.001	94	7	10	.673	.001	86	5	14

Note. ChIPS = Children's Interview for Psychiatric Syndromes. DICA-R-C = DSM-III-R–revised Diagnostic Interview for Children and Adolescents.

[a]Low-base-rate kappa (κ_x) was used when there was less than 25% endorsement on both the ChIPS and the DICA-R-C, as indicated with footnote.

[b]Number of cases in which the syndrome was scored as present by both interviews.

[c]Number of cases in which the syndrome was scored as absent by both interviews.

[d]Kappa coefficients could not be determined for these syndromes because of 100% agreement on their absence.

Table 10. Agreement on Syndrome Endorsement Between the ChIPS and the DICA-R-C: Study IV (21 Child [Ages 6 to 12 Years] and 19 Adolescent [Ages 13 to 17 Years] Psychiatric Inpatients)

Syndrome	Children					Adolescents				
	κ^a	$P <$	Agreement (%)	Yes/Yes[b]	No/No[c]	κ^a	$P <$	Agreement (%)	Yes/Yes[b]	No/No[c]
Attention-deficit/hyperactivity disorder	.422	.024	71	6	9	.568[a]	.010	84	1	15
Oppositional defiant disorder	.493	.009	86	10	8	.481	.014	89	9	8
Conduct disorder	.712	.001	76	11	5	.791	.001	74	6	8
Substance abuse	—[d]	—	100	0	21	.627[a]	.02	63	1	16
Simple phobia	.811[a]	.010	95	2	18	.525[a]	.006	79	1	14
Social phobia	.488[a]	.156	95	0	20	.747[a]	.002	89	3	14
Separation anxiety disorder	.625[a]	.001	81	3	14	.532[a]	.002	74	2	12
Generalized anxiety disorder	.475[a]	.075	90	0	19	.532[a]	.002	74	2	12
Obsessive-compulsive disorder	—[d]	—	100	0	21	.486[a]	.156	95	0	18
Posttraumatic stress disorder	1.00[a]	.074	100	1	20	.672[a]	.001	84	3	13
Anorexia	—[d]	—	100	0	21	—[d]	—	100	0	19
Bulimia	—[d]	—	100	0	21	—[d]	—	100	0	19
Major depressive disorder	.667	.001	86	5	13	.379	.037	74	11	3
Dysthymic disorder	1.00[a]	.001	100	4	17	.582	.005	79	8	7
Manic episode	.475[a]	.075	90	0	19	.472[a]	.074	89	0	17
Enuresis	.850[a]	.003	95	3	17	—[d]	—	100	1	18
Encopresis	—[d]	—	100	0	21	.486[a]	.156	95	0	18
Psychosis	.889	.001	95	6	14	.671	.002	84	6	10

Note. ChIPS = Children's Interview for Psychiatric Syndromes. DICA-R-C = DSM-III-R–revised Diagnostic Interview for Children and Adolescents.

[a]Low-base-rate kappa (κ_x) was used when there was less than 25% endorsement on both the ChIPS and the DICA-R-C, as indicated with footnote.

[b]Number of cases in which the syndrome was scored as present by both interviews.

[c]Number of cases in which the syndrome was scored as absent by both interviews.

[d]Kappa coefficients could not be determined for these syndromes because of 100% agreement on their absence.

Table 11. Agreement on Syndrome Endorsement Between the ChIPS and the DICA-R-C: Study V (40 Community-Based Children and Adolescents Ages 6 to 18 Years)

Syndrome	κ[a]	$P <$	Agreement (%)	Yes/Yes[b]	No/No[c]
Attention-deficit/hyperactivity disorder	.494	.16	97.5	0	39
Oppositional defiant disorder	—[d]	—	100	0	40
Conduct disorder	1.00	.08	100	1	39
Alcohol abuse	—[d]	—	100	0	40
Cigarette abuse	.494	.16	97.5	0	39
Drug abuse	—[d]	—	100	0	40
Simple phobia	.478	.001	77.5	1	30
Social phobia	.494	.16	97.5	0	39
Separation anxiety disorder	.487	.08	95	0	38
Generalized anxiety disorder	.487	.08	95	0	38
Obsessive-compulsive disorder	—[d]	—	100	0	40
Posttraumatic stress disorder	—[d]	—	100	0	40
Anorexia	—[d]	—	100	0	40
Bulimia	—[d]	—	100	0	40
Major depressive disorder	—[d]	—	100	0	40
Dysthymic disorder	—[d]	—	100	0	40
Manic episode	—[d]	—	100	0	40
Enuresis	1.00	.08	100	1	39
Encopresis	—[d]	—	100	0	40
Psychosis	—[d]	—	100	0	40

Note. ChIPS = Children's Interview for Psychiatric Syndromes. DICA-R-C = DSM-III-R–revised Diagnostic Interview for Children and Adolescents.

[a]Low-base-rate kappa (κ_x) was used.

[b]Number of cases in which the syndrome was scored as present by both interviews.

[c]Number of cases in which the syndrome was scored as absent by both interviews.

[d]Kappa coefficients could not be determined for these syndromes because of 100% agreement on their absence.

Table 12.   Agreement on Symptom Endorsement Between the ChIPS and the DICA-R-C: Study V (40 Community-Based Children and Adolescents Ages 6 to 18 Years)

Syndrome	κ^a	$P <$	Agreement (%)	Yes/Yes[b]	No/No[c]
Attention-deficit/hyperactivity disorder	.451	.001	65	3	23
Oppositional defiant disorder	.453	.001	72.5	1	28
Conduct disorder	.568	.006	90	1	35
Alcohol abuse	.481	.04	92.5	0	37
Cigarette abuse	.822	.01	97.5	2	37
Drug abuse	.494	.16	97.5	0	39
Simple phobia	.615	.001	77.5	8	23
Social phobia	.494	.16	97.5	0	39
Separation anxiety disorder	.494	.001	87.5	3	32
Generalized anxiety disorder	.822	.01	97.5	2	37
Obsessive-compulsive disorder	—[d]	—	100	0	40
Posttraumatic stress disorder	—[d]	—	100	0	40
Anorexia	.474	.02	90	0	36
Bulimia	.494	.16	97.5	0	39
Major depressive disorder	.524	.002	85	1	33
Dysthymic disorder	.487	.08	95	0	38
Manic episode	—[d]	—	100	0	40
Enuresis	.474	.02	90	1	35
Encopresis	.494	.16	97.5	0	39
Psychosis	.341	.08	95	0	38

Note.   ChIPS = Children's Interview for Psychiatric Syndromes. DICA-R-C = DSM-III-R–revised Diagnostic Interview for Children and Adolescents.

[a]Low-base-rate kappa (κ_x) was used.

[b]Number of cases in which the syndrome was scored as present by both interviews.

[c]Number of cases in which the syndrome was scored as absent by both interviews.

[d]Kappa coefficients could not be determined for these syndromes because of 100% agreement on their absence.

Table 13. Agreement on Syndrome Endorsement Between the ChIPS and the Consensus Panel: Study V (40 Community-Based Children and Adolescents Ages 6 to 18 Years)

Syndrome	κ[a]	$P <$	Agreement (%)	Yes/Yes[b]	No/No[c]
Attention-deficit/hyperactivity disorder	1.00	.08	100	1	39
Oppositional defiant disorder	.494	.16	97.5	0	39
Conduct disorder	1.00	.16	100	1	39
Alcohol abuse	—[d]	—	100	0	40
Cigarette abuse	.494	.16	97.5	0	39
Drug abuse	—[d]	—	100	0	40
Simple phobia	.453	.001	72.5	1	28
Social phobia	.494	.16	97.5	0	39
Separation anxiety disorder	.487	.08	95	0	38
Generalized anxiety disorder	.740	.04	97.5	1	38
Obsessive-compulsive disorder	—[d]	—	100	0	40
Posttraumatic stress disorder	—[d]	—	100	0	40
Anorexia	—[d]	—	100	0	40
Bulimia	—[d]	—	100	0	40
Major depressive disorder	—[d]	—	100	0	40
Dysthymic disorder	.494	.16	97.5	0	39
Manic episode	—[d]	—	100	0	40
Enuresis	1.00	.08	100	1	39
Encopresis	—[d]	—	100	0	40
Psychosis	—[d]	—	100	0	40

Note. ChIPS = Children's Interview for Psychiatric Syndromes.

[a]Low-base-rate kappa (κ_x) was used.

[b]Number of cases in which the syndrome was scored as present by both interviews.

[c]Number of cases in which the syndrome was scored as absent by both interviews.

[d]Kappa coefficients could not be determined for these syndromes because of 100% agreement on their absence.

Table 14. Agreement on Symptom Endorsement Between the ChIPS and the Consensus Panel: Study V (40 Community-Based Children and Adolescents Ages 6 to 18 Years)

Syndrome	κ[a]	$P <$	Agreement (%)	Yes/Yes[b]	No/No[c]
Attention-deficit/hyperactivity disorder	.398	.001	55	5	17
Oppositional defiant disorder	.464	.001	65	4	22
Conduct disorder	.568	.006	90	1	35
Alcohol abuse	.481	.04	92.5	0	37
Cigarette abuse	.822	.01	97.5	2	37
Drug abuse	.494	.16	97.5	0	39
Simple phobia	.588	.001	75	8	22
Social phobia	.494	.16	97.5	0	39
Separation anxiety disorder	.638	.001	87.5	3	32
Generalized anxiety disorder	.778	.002	95	3	35
Obsessive-compulsive disorder	—[d]	—	100	0	40
Posttraumatic stress disorder	—[d]	—	100	0	40
Anorexia	.474	.02	90	0	36
Bulimia	.494	.16	97.5	0	39
Major depressive disorder	.512	.001	77.5	2	29
Dysthymic disorder	.543	.003	87.5	1	34
Manic episode	—[d]	—	100	0	40
Enuresis	.568	.006	90	1	35
Encopresis	.491	.16	97.5	0	39
Psychosis	.481	.04	92.5	0	37

Note. ChIPS = Children's Interview for Psychiatric Syndromes.

[a]Low-base-rate kappa (κ_x) was used.

[b]Number of cases in which the syndrome was scored as present by both interviews.

[c]Number of cases in which the syndrome was scored as absent by both interviews.

[d]Kappa coefficients could not be determined for these syndromes because of 100% agreement on their absence.

Chapter 6: Interpretations and Case Examples

All of the cases described in this chapter are taken from actual ChIPS interviews. Names and other identifying information have been altered to protect the child's confidentiality.

Case Report 1

Gary is a 10-year-old male presenting to an inpatient child psychiatric facility. When asked why he was admitted, he stated, "I'm sick. I've been having headaches from my medicine, and my behavior has been bad." The medicine he was currently taking was Ritalin (methylphenidate).

Behavioral Observations

Gary was neatly groomed and dressed. During the first 15 minutes of the interview he cried, saying he wanted his mother. He talked at length about how he missed his mother and how he wanted to leave to be with her. After some reassurance, Gary calmed down enough to continue with the interview. He was cooperative and displayed good effort when not preoccupied with his separation from his mother.

ChIPS Results

Gary fulfilled ChIPS diagnostic criteria for Oppositional Defiant Disorder, Conduct Disorder, Separation Anxiety Disorder, and Enuresis.

Gary was not sure when his oppositional symptoms began, but he knew it was at least several years ago. These symptoms included refusing to do what his parents asked him to do; finding that other people made him mad all the time; and becoming easily angered by others. He also reported getting even with people who made him mad by doing something wrong and then blaming it on them.

Gary's conduct became a problem when he was 6 years old. He began stealing toys and candy from stores. He also said he "goes off" without any reason and gets into fights. In the days prior to admission he threatened his mother with a butcher knife during an argument. He dented his grandmother's car when she told Gary's mother about something he had done wrong. Currently he was participating in a fire setter's program because of his history of setting fires. He also acknowledged having forced someone to play with his private parts, but said he could not remember who this was.

Under Separation Anxiety Disorder, Gary endorsed all eight symptoms. He begs his mother to stay home whenever she leaves the house, because he is afraid she will get into an automobile accident. He also worries about her getting sick. When he is not with his parents, he is afraid that he will die and never see them again. When he goes to school, he worries about his mother and cries; however, he said his Ritalin was helping him with this. Additionally, he reported following his mother around at home, not being able to sleep without his mother, having bad dreams about his mother dying, and experiencing headaches when he has to leave home to go to school. These worries began when Gary was in first grade and continue to cause problems for him.

Gary was unsure of when his enuretic symptoms started. It was apparent that they have lasted more than 3 months, however. He wets the bed almost every night but does not wet himself during the day.

The only other symptoms Gary endorsed were those of Attention-Deficit/Hyperactivity Disorder. Although he endorsed several inattentive and hyperactive symptoms, they were insufficient in number to qualify him for a diagnosis. Gary was taking Ritalin for these problems, and the staff's observations during the course of his stay included behaviors such as interruptions in class and an inability both to stay focused on the task at hand and to sit quietly.

Clinician's Diagnosis

On discharge, Gary's clinical diagnoses included Attention-Deficit/Hyperactivity Disorder, Combined type; Conduct Disorder; and Separation Anxiety Disorder. During his stay, Gary was started on imipramine, and his enuresis resolved.

Comment

Gary qualified for diagnoses of Oppositional Defiant Disorder and Conduct Disorder according to ChIPS criteria. Rarely would a child in a clinical situation be diagnosed with both disorders, however. Although these are separate disorders and have distinct features, they are best viewed as existing on a continuum. Conduct Disorder is characterized by behavior that violates age-appropriate social norms and the rights of others. It is more severe than the excessive defiance toward authority figures exhibited by a child with Oppositional Defiant Disorder. When a child meets criteria for both disorders, Conduct Disorder is diagnosed because it is considered the more inclusive diagnosis. The ChIPS is not designed to make this distinction; rather, it is intended to assess childhood psychiatric syndromes at the individual level. The clinician must use this information to determine the appropriate diagnosis for the child. For these reasons, Gary received only the diagnosis of Conduct Disorder, not of Oppositional Defiant Disorder.

Gary endorsed symptoms of Attention-Deficit/Hyperactivity Disorder; however, these were of insufficient quantity to result in his meeting diagnostic criteria. This finding frequently occurs in partially treated children and highlights the need to receive collateral information from parents and teachers as well as to integrate knowledge of current treatment (i.e., he is currently taking Ritalin) when deriving a clinical diagnosis.

Case Report 2

Tamara is a 12-year-old female presenting to an inpatient child psychiatric facility. When asked why she was admitted, she stated that she was getting into fights with her family and other kids at school.

Behavioral Observations

Tamara was neatly dressed. Her mood was slightly euphoric. She was extremely talkative throughout the interview and was quite tangential. She giggled at many questions, and there were many questions that had to be explained or repeated because Tamara either misunderstood or did not hear them. She responded well to redirection and was cooperative throughout the interview.

ChIPS Results

Tamara fulfilled ChIPS diagnostic criteria for Attention-Deficit/Hyperactivity Disorder, Oppositional Defiant Disorder, Conduct Disorder, Mania, and Psychosis.

She reported Attention-Deficit/Hyperactivity Disorder symptoms but could not recall when they first began. She said that they were "always there." Tamara reported the following symptoms of inattention: having trouble keeping her mind on what she is doing; being told by her parents that she does not listen to them; frequently going from one thing to another without finishing anything; and having difficulty sticking to what she is doing when other things are going on around her. She also endorsed symptoms of hyperactivity. These included often being told to sit still; having difficulty staying in her seat; getting in trouble for running around at home and school; getting in trouble for being too loud when she plays; being told by her parents that she is always "on the go"; getting in trouble for talking too much at home; blurting out answers to questions before they have been completed; and interrupting others when they are doing things. Tamara qualified for a diagnosis of Attention-Deficit/Hyperactivity Disorder, Hyperactive–Impulsive type.

Tamara also reported that her oppositional symptoms had always been present. She reported losing her temper a lot, often arguing with her parents, refusing to do what her parents and teachers asked of her, doing things on purpose to bug other people, and blaming other people for her own mistakes. She also said that it was easy for other people to make her mad, and that when they did, she usually got even by starting a fight.

Just as she had reported regarding her symptoms of Attention-Deficit/Hyperactivity Disorder and Oppositional Defiant Disorder, Tamara stated that her conduct symptoms were "always there." She endorsed lying to get out of things she doesn't want to do, threatening other people, and often being involved in fights.

Although Tamara's manic symptoms had been present for as long as she could remember, she stated that they had become a real problem only recently. She endorsed feelings of extreme cheerfulness and also feelings of irritability. According to her, these feelings were present in her life even in the absence of any precipitating events. Tamara also reported having a lot of energy and not needing sleep, speaking very fast and talking without being able to be stopped, having racing thoughts, having trouble keeping her mind on what she is doing without being distracted, having a lot more energy than usual, and getting hurt because she is not careful. These symptoms were directly related to the problems that brought her to the hospital.

Tamara's symptoms of psychosis began when she was 6 years old. They included auditory and visual hallucinations that occurred only upon falling asleep, not during the daytime. She had visions of deceased family members coming out of their graves and holding bloody hearts. Tamara also had been hearing voices telling her that "they" are going to kill her brother, sister, and parents. Since she has been having these experiences, she has had difficulty in her interpersonal relationships. She has lost friends, and life at home has been difficult. Although the visions and voices have lasted on and off for more than 6 months, the active psychotic features were not present for most of the past month. Tamara thus met the Duration criteria for Psychosis rather than for Schizophrenia.

The only other symptoms Tamara endorsed were those of Major Depressive Disorder. She reported hating herself, and said that she "can't achieve anything." She also said she wishes she had not been born and sometimes thinks about suicide. Recently, these symptoms have become more pervasive in association with Tamara's manic and psychotic symptoms. Although her depressive symptoms were serious, they did not in themselves qualify for a diagnosis of Major Depressive Disorder.

Clinician's Diagnosis

Upon discharge, Tamara received the diagnosis of Bipolar I Disorder, most recent episode manic, with psychotic features.

Comment

This case illustrates an important point concerning the proper use and interpretation of the ChIPS. The ChIPS is to be used as an assessment tool. It screens for symptom clusters in areas that are problematic for many children and adolescents. It is not a replacement for clinical judgment and experience. The child with overlapping symptomatology of multiple disorders presents a clinical dilemma. The clinician must ascertain whether the symptoms warrant diagnoses of multiple disorders or whether they are features of a single disorder. Because of its nonhierarchical nature, the ChIPS is not designed to make this distinction. It is, however, possible to compare the ages at onset of the disorders in question to determine whether they originated at the same point in time. If they did, there is an increased likelihood that the symptoms derive from one primary disorder. In Tamara's case, ChIPS results included Attention-Deficit/Hyperactivity Disorder, Oppositional Defiant Disorder, Conduct Disorder, Mania, and Psychosis. When the ages at onset of these various diagnoses were compared, it was found that Tamara's problems began at the same time. The only diagnosis with a different age at onset was Psychosis, which began when Tamara was 6 years old. In addition, her symptoms for the various disorders overlapped and were dominated by features of irritability and hyperactivity.

Tamara's parents reported a recent decline in her functioning at home and school. Three weeks prior to her admission, Tamara had developed symptoms of a viral illness, including vomiting, nausea, and diarrhea. Although she recovered from these, her behavioral symptoms began soon after. Her parents noticed that she was abnormally quiet for 3 or 4 days and then began showing signs of hyperactivity. She talked non-stop and refused to listen to her parents. She had been an honor roll student for the past 2 years but now began to struggle with schoolwork. She also began to threaten schoolmates and family members and became involved in fights. During this period, she received her first detention at school. Prior to admission, Tamara's parents also found her up late drawing pictures and symbols on her body. Although Tamara reported having heard voices since first grade, neither her parents nor her teachers reported any abnormal behavior before this episode. The fact that her symptoms began at the same time and shared common features makes it likely that they are all the manifestation of a primary condition, in this case Bipolar Disorder. The clinician examining Tamara used hierarchical decision making to arrive at this conclusion.

Case Report 3

Bobby is an 11-year-old male presenting to an inpatient child psychiatric facility. When asked why he was admitted, he explained that he had been burned by a smoke bomb that exploded while he was making it.

Behavioral Observations

Bobby was neatly dressed. His face was red from the burns he had sustained prior to admission. He also had many scrapes and scars on his arms and legs that he reported were from careless accidents. Bobby was very talkative and often recounted stories unrelated to the questions asked. He was easily redirected, however, and cooperated throughout the interview.

ChIPS Results

Bobby fulfilled ChIPS diagnostic criteria for Attention-Deficit/Hyperactivity Disorder, Oppositional Defiant Disorder, and Conduct Disorder.

He reported Attention-Deficit/Hyperactivity Disorder symptoms with an onset at age 6. Bobby endorsed the following symptoms of inattention: making lots of careless mistakes on his schoolwork; having trouble keeping his mind on what he is doing; being told by his parents that he is not listening; starting his schoolwork and not finishing it; avoiding his schoolwork; losing things like papers a lot; and having trouble sticking to what he is doing when other things are going on around him. He also acknowledged symptoms of hyperactivity. These included being told to sit still a lot; having trouble staying in his seat; having a difficult time playing quietly; being told by his parents that he is always "on the go"; blurting out answers to questions before they have been completed; and interrupting other people when they are doing things. Bobby qualified for a diagnosis of Attention-Deficit/Hyperactivity Disorder, Combined type.

Bobby reported that his oppositional symptoms began when he was 7. He reported throwing temper tantrums often, talking back to his parents a lot, breaking rules at home, doing things on purpose to bug other people, blaming his mistakes on others, finding that other people make him mad all the time, finding it easy for other people to make him mad, and getting even with people who make him mad. These problems caused him considerable trouble and were more than expected for his age.

Bobby reported that his symptoms of Conduct Disorder first appeared when he was 4 years old. He indicated that he often lied to get out of doing schoolwork and household chores. He said he often stays out later than his parents say he can. He has been in trouble for fighting and has used weapons in fights, including a chain and a pellet gun. His fighting has resulted in injury to others. Bobby reported stealing a nightstick and bashing in neighborhood cars. He also endorsed fire setting. For instance, he made "jellied gasoline that was like napalm" with his chemistry set and set his driveway on fire.

The only other symptoms on the ChIPS endorsed by Bobby were those of Major Depressive Disorder, including irritable mood, having difficulty falling asleep, and being unable to sit still when he is feeling irritable, but there were not enough of these symptoms to merit the diagnosis.

Clinician's Diagnosis

Upon discharge, Bobby was given clinical diagnoses of Attention-Deficit/Hyperactivity Disorder, Combined type, and Conduct Disorder.

Case Report 4

Diane is a thin, 16-year-old female presenting to an inpatient psychiatric facility. When asked why she was admitted, she said she was always tired, was unable to think straight, and was thinking about killing herself.

Behavioral Observations

Diane was visibly upset during the initial interview. She repeatedly stated that she wanted to go home and seemed on the verge of crying. With reassurance she was able to continue, but only for short periods of time. She stared blankly and made minimal eye contact. Her answers were slow, and questions had to be asked multiple times. When she did answer, there was no emotion in her voice, and it was questionable whether she was understanding the questions. After 15 minutes, it was apparent that Diane was not capable of reliably completing the interview, and the interview was terminated. Five days later, after Diane was stabilized on medication, the interview was attempted again. She seemed much improved. Diane was more attentive and less upset, although psychomotor retardation was still noted. She also exhibited inappropriate smiling and said that she could not stop herself from smiling. Diane yawned often and appeared to be sleepy during parts of the interview. Midway through this second interview, the interviewer suggested taking a break, which appeared to be helpful. Diane's attention was focused when the interview resumed. She was able to complete the second interview and appeared to understand the questions.

ChIPS Results

Diane fulfilled ChIPS diagnostic criteria for Major Depressive Disorder, Dysthymic Disorder, and Psychosis.

Diane said that her depressive symptoms had begun when she was 14. She reported having felt sad and mad almost every day since then. She also noted that it sometimes seemed that every day was the same day occurring over and over again. Diane acknowledged feeling left out and unable to have fun. For the past 2 years, Diane reported lacking energy and having bad thoughts about herself. She thinks she is "ugly, stupid, and retarded." Over the past year, she has not been able to remember things as well as usual. She has felt hopeless and in the past few weeks has wished she were dead. During this time, she tried to kill herself by putting a knife to her stomach. She still has these feelings of wanting to kill herself. When asked whether she had any plans about how she would do this, she replied that she would eat the hospital food, which was poisoned.

Additionally, Diane believed that the nurses and doctors spied on her and were trying to kill her. She reported visual hallucinations that occurred upon falling asleep. These consisted of seeing ghosts, but Diane's description was vague, and she was unable to give any additional details about this experience. Auditory hallucinations were denied. Since her problems had started, she admitted to having less friends and being less careful about her looks. To her best recollection, these psychotic symptoms began when she was 11 but have been worse in the past month.

Clinician's Diagnosis

On discharge, Diane was diagnosed with Major Depressive Disorder, recurrent with psychotic features, and a rule-out diagnosis of Schizoaffective Disorder.

Comment

This case illustrates the importance of gathering information from as many sources as possible before making a diagnosis. In Diane's case, the question was whether she had Major Depressive Disorder with psychotic features or Schizoaffective Disorder. This distinction was important for both therapeutic and prognostic reasons. On the ChIPS, Diane endorsed depression beginning at age 14 and psychosis beginning at age 11 years. This leads one to suspect that Diane has Schizoaffective Disorder, since the psychotic features were present before any depressive symptoms. To help clarify the situation, Diane's parents were interviewed; however, it was found that they were largely unaware of her problems. They had knowledge of her depressive symptoms but were not aware of the psychosis until the hospital staff informed them upon Diane's admission. During the ChIPS interview, Diane reported that her parents ignored her a lot. In light of this, it was perhaps not surprising that Diane was referred to the emergency room by her school nurse rather than her family. Because she had not been a troublemaker at school, however, she had only recently come to the attention of school authorities. Diane presented a difficult clinical diagnostic situation. Only after consideration of all available information was Diane's diagnosis able to be determined.

Case Report 5

Doug is a 16-year-old male presenting to an inpatient psychiatric facility. When asked what problems he was having, he said he had "suicidal tendencies." He had tried to cut his arm with a screwdriver after an argument with his mother. He also reported disliking school because of all the "preps, jocks, and snobs" there. Additionally, he said he did not have any real friends. Doug noted that he is not allowed to be around the other kids in his neighborhood because their parents think he is a bad influence.

Behavioral Observations

Doug appeared disheveled, and his clothing was frayed. Throughout the interview, he bit at his sleeves and pulled on his clothes. He had lacerations on his forearms that he said were from razor blades. His affect was flat, and he lacked energy. He spoke in a low monotone and at times was difficult to understand. Nevertheless, Doug was cooperative and displayed good attention during the course of the interview.

ChIPS Results

Doug fulfilled ChIPS diagnostic criteria for Conduct Disorder, Substance Abuse–Nicotine, Major Depressive Disorder, and Dysthymic Disorder.

Doug could not remember at what age his conduct symptoms began. He did, however, remember trying to put the family cat in the microwave when he was very young (i.e., preschool). That was his earliest recollection of symptoms. Other conduct symptoms included stealing from family members; lying to get out of doing things; and damaging property. In the 2 weeks preceding his admission, he was suspended from school twice for vandalizing school property.

Doug reported beginning to abuse substances at age 13, when he started to smoke cigarettes and marijuana. He had smoked marijuana three times per week for a period of 2 months but had stopped when he was 14. He continues to smoke half a pack of cigarettes per day even though he has been suspended from school and grounded because of his smoking. This impairment from cigarette smoking fulfilled criteria for substance abuse. Because Doug reported no impairment related to marijuana, and he had stopped using it 2 years ago, his use of that substance did not fulfill criteria for abuse.

Doug's depressive symptoms began when he was 12. He endorsed feelings of sadness that have been present for more days than not over the past 4 years. In the past month, this dysphoria has been much harder to deal with and has occurred more frequently, almost every day. When asked what he has fun doing, he explained that he enjoyed playing the guitar, singing, and writing songs. This response was given with no enthusiasm, in a flat monotone. He reported no other interests. He appeared to have a fascination with a popular rock musician and spontaneously brought up the musician's name in conversation. Doug stated that the only thing that cheers him up is talking to pictures of this musician that he has placed all over his bedroom walls. Interestingly, the musician in question committed suicide 2 years ago. When asked about his sleep habits, Doug said that he was often sleepy and took naps during the day. These sleep problems have been present on and off for the past few years but have been an everyday occurrence in the past month. Doug also admitted to having bad thoughts about himself; he said he was a loser and could not do anything right. When he had these thoughts, he would mutilate his arm with a razor blade. He also had recently attempted suicide by trying to cut his throat with a pair of scissors.

Doug endorsed several inattention symptoms of Attention-Deficit/Hyperactivity Disorder and reported having taken Ritalin since childhood to control these problems. He did not, however, endorse enough symptoms to qualify for a diagnosis. The only other symptoms endorsed were those of Oppositional Defiant Disorder.

Clinician's Diagnosis

Doug was discharged with the diagnoses of Major Depressive Disorder, Dysthymic Disorder, Conduct Disorder, and Attention-Deficit/Hyperactivity Disorder.

Case Report 6

Lauren is a 16-year-old female participating in a child bereavement study 13 months after her father's death.

Behavioral Observations

Lauren was neatly dressed for the interview and appeared mature for her age. She was open, friendly, and cooperative throughout the interview.

ChIPS Results

Lauren fulfilled ChIPS diagnostic criteria for Generalized Anxiety Disorder. She endorsed worrying more than other kids her age; in fact, she said she worries every day. She described worrying about where she will go to college, how she will pay for college, and what she will do when she grows up. Although these are not unusual concerns for someone of her age, Lauren reported that when she worries it is hard for her to calm down and relax and that she tends to get cranky easily. She also stated that her muscles get tight and she gets headaches when she worries. When asked how long she has worried like this, Lauren said, "Always"; however, she did not believe that these worries caused her problems at home, at school, or with peers.

Lauren also endorsed several symptoms of Attention-Deficit/Hyperactivity Disorder, Oppositional Defiant Disorder, and Separation Anxiety Disorder. However, the number of endorsements were insufficient to make any diagnoses.

Clinician's Diagnosis

Lauren was given a diagnosis of Generalized Anxiety Disorder by the consensus panel research team.

Comment

This case illustrates how clinicians must judiciously use the Impairment criteria in the ChIPS. Lauren described anxiety about commonplace events, but this anxiety resulted in somatic complaints and generalized feelings of tension and irritability. When asked about any interference these symptoms caused at home, school, or with peers, Lauren denied that there was a problem, but later in the interview, she admitted going to see her school counselor on a regular basis to discuss her concerns and worries.

Case Report 7

Alex is a 10-year-old male participating in a research study as a community comparison subject.

Behavioral Observations

Alex was outgoing and talkative throughout the interview.

ChIPS Results

Alex fulfilled ChIPS diagnostic criteria for Enuresis. He endorsed still wetting the bed at night and said that this happens even when he is not sick. Alex reported that he has been wetting the bed for as long as he can remember, and that it typically happens three times per week.

Alex also endorsed several symptoms of Attention-Deficit/Hyperactivity Disorder and Oppositional Defiant Disorder. However, the number of endorsements made were insufficient to warrant a diagnosis.

Clinician's Diagnosis

Upon consensus panel review, Alex was given a diagnosis of Enuresis.

Chapter 7: Training

This chapter provides complete specifications for training mental health professionals and paraprofessionals to administer the ChIPS. Training can occur individually or in groups. The discussion below is presented for training in a group format. Individual training can proceed in the same manner, with discussion being limited to one trainee and one trainer.

Step 1. Familiarization

Step 1 involves familiarizing trainees with the interview procedure and with childhood psychopathology in general. Trainees are given a copy of the interview, the scoring form, and this manual, with the instructions to study them thoroughly and to write down any questions or concerns. Additionally, trainees are asked to read pertinent sections from DSM-IV (American Psychiatric Association 1994; i.e., Disorders Usually First Diagnosed in Infancy, Childhood, and Adolescence; Mood Disorders; Anxiety Disorders; Eating Disorders; Schizophrenia and Other Psychotic Disorders) to develop an awareness of the clinical conditions they will be assessing. Group discussion (reviewed in steps 2 and 3 below) will allow trainees to raise questions regarding their understanding of the interview and the scoring form and about child and adolescent symptomatology.

Step 2. Review of General Interviewing Procedures

The next step in the training process involves a group discussion of the entire interview. Topics to be discussed are reviewed below; they include initially meeting the child; conducting a thorough interview; handling "if yes" and "if no" statements; when to ask Duration questions; and how to ask Duration questions. Throughout the familiarization process, any additional questions or concerns of trainees should be addressed.

Initially meeting the child.   The first impression an interviewer makes on a child may significantly affect the interview's validity. First, the interviewer should introduce him- or herself to the child and briefly explain the testing procedure. The interviewer should attempt to establish an alliance with the child at this point in the interaction. Because the child may not initially be interested in being interviewed, the interviewer will probably increase the chances of success by developing good rapport with the child and obtaining the child's assent prior to the interview. Introductory comments and general questions about the presenting problem, family, school, and friends that appear on the first page of the instrument are designed, in part, to help the interviewer get a general "feel" for the child and for the important aspects of his or her life.

The child should be encouraged to inform the interviewer if he or she does not understand a question. For example, the interviewer might say "Lots of boys/girls/teenagers your age don't always understand the questions I'm about to ask. If that happens to you, make sure to stop me and have me explain better, okay?" It is also good to include a statement explaining the general nature of the questions to the child. For example, "Some of the questions I'm going to ask you will fit you pretty well. Other questions won't fit you at all. My job is to ask all the questions, so we can see which ones fit and which ones don't."

Conducting a thorough interview.   The ChIPS is a screening interview, meaning that it explores the possible occurrence of 20 syndromes in children. If there is a judgment call regarding whether to ask or skip the remaining questions in a section, the questions should be asked. If an error is to be made, it should be on the side of being too inclusive rather than too exclusive. For example, a child who appears anxious or depressed or whose parent reports the chief complaint to be "My child looks sad and worried all the time" should be asked *all* of the questions listed under Generalized Anxiety Disorder and Depression/Dysthymia, even if the child denies the symptoms covered in the cardinal questions. This allows the child to either confirm or deny other symptoms. If subsequent questions were not asked, such an opportunity would not exist. If the child answers a sufficient amount of questions in a section positively, the interviewer should return and repeat questions previously denied from the beginning of the section. It may be that after feeling more comfortable admitting to symptoms, the child can more honestly answer the initial questions.

Handling "if yes" statements.   Statements such as "if yes" appear throughout the interview. These statements are included to expedite the interview process.

Example from Oppositional Defiant Disorder section:

1.   a)   **Do you usually get upset and lose your temper if things don't go your way?** If yes, go
            to 2.
     b)   **Do you throw big temper tantrums pretty often?**

The phrase "if yes, go to 2" is included because if the child answers in the affirmative, he or she meets that criterion. No other information is required. The interviewer skips 1b and proceeds to 2. Again, if an error in using "if yes" questions is made, it should be made in asking too many, rather than too few, questions.

Handling "if no" statements.   Statements such as "if no" also appear throughout the interview. These statements keep the interviewer from asking unnecessary questions.

Example from Mania/Hypomania section:

1.   a)   **Are there times when you feel *very, very good*, on top of the world, like you could do
            anything? or like everything is wonderful?** If yes, have child describe. If no, go to 2.

This skip keeps the interviewer from asking the child more questions about a euphoric mood that, if the child answered "no," did not occur.

When to ask Duration questions.   The Duration questions should be asked when the preceding criteria have been met. For example, in the Oppositional Defiant Disorder section, if four or more of the numbered questions have an affirmative response, the Duration section would be administered. If the child has not met the specified criteria, these questions would not be asked.

How to ask Duration questions.   Time and duration are often difficult concepts for children, especially young children. It is particularly useful to develop a framework for time intervals that are relevant to each child (e.g., "from the end of last school year until now," "from Christmas until your birthday") to use when asking Duration questions. However, there may be times when it is nearly impossible to determine the duration of a particular disorder. It may also become obvious during an interview that, regardless of disorder, the child will not be able to provide duration details, either because the child's sense of time is not well enough developed or because the child cannot remember the events in question. To provide for such an eventuality, the ChIPS scoring form contains separate places for 1) noting when symptom criteria (excluding duration) have been met and 2) recording Duration criteria for each disorder.

An example of how such a situation might be handled follows. A child is interviewed and meets criteria for Separation Anxiety Disorder. The interviewer asks the Duration questions, to which the child responds, "I don't know." Further explanation of the Duration criteria (e.g., since Christmas, summer, your birthday) does not help. In an attempt to provide the necessary structure for the concept of the "4 weeks" criterion, the child is asked to say the days of the week but cannot give the names in the right order. It is thus apparent that the child's conceptualization of time is not well enough developed to allow an accurate response. The interviewer would mark the box indicating that symptom criteria are met but should *not* mark the box indicating that Duration criteria have been met.

Although it is generally true that a child who cannot answer Duration questions for one disorder cannot answer them for any disorder, this is not always the case. Duration questions should be attempted at least several times, until the interviewer is convinced that the child's inability to specify duration is not syndrome specific. For example, a child with a long-standing disorder may not know when it started or how long it has gone on but may be able to provide information about syndromes with a more recent onset. Any uncertainty the interviewer has about the child's ability to conceptualize and accurately report on time should be noted in the Behavioral Observations section on the profile sheet of the scoring form.

How to count endorsements. ChIPS is designed to provide alternative wording for many symptom queries. These take the form of subparts to the questions (e.g., 1a, 1b, 1c). Once a symptom is endorsed, however, the interviewer proceeds to the next numeric question. Thus, when scoring criteria require a certain number (e.g., three) of questions to be endorsed, this requirement refers to the quantity of *numbered* questions endorsed rather than to the quantity of question subparts endorsed (i.e., if three endorsements are required, endorsement of questions 1a, 1b, and 2 would not count, whereas endorsement of questions 1, 2, and 4 would).

Step 3. Review of Specific Disorders

After reviewing general principles of testing, a group discussion of each specific disorder covered in the ChIPS should be held. The material presented below should be addressed in this discussion.

Attention-Deficit/Hyperactivity Disorder. Attention-Deficit/Hyperactivity Disorder requires six or more symptoms to be endorsed in either of two sections, Inattention and Hyperactivity–Impulsivity. This section begins with a preface, a probe, and a note.

> **Preface**
>
> **Sometimes children/teenagers behave in a way that causes problems at home or at school. I'm going to ask you about some problems, and I want you to tell me if they have ever happened to you.**
>
> **Probe**
>
> If child says "sometimes" or is equivocal about an answer, ask: **Has that happened so much that it caused you problems at home or at school, like getting yelled at a lot or punished?**
>
> **Note:** Score only if behavior occurs more often than in other children/teenagers of same age.

The purpose of the preface is to introduce the child to the entire interview. The probe and note aid the interviewer in making the distinction between normal inattention and restlessness and that which crosses the border into symptomatic behavior.

Another item to note in the Attention-Deficit/Hyperactivity Disorder section is found in Section B, Question 7:

> 7. **Do you often blurt out answers to questions before they have been completed?** (Rate as "yes" if this occurs during the interview, even if the child says "no.")

The purpose of this note is to allow the interviewer to use personal observation of symptoms exhibited during the interview. It should be noted on the profile sheet of the scoring form if the child denies a symptom that is observed by the interviewer.

Oppositional Defiant Disorder. Oppositional Defiant Disorder requires endorsement of at least four of the eight numbered questions. For example, if the only positive endorsements were 3a, 3b, 3c, and 4, the child would not qualify for this disorder, because only two of the numbered questions have been endorsed. If, however, 1a, 2b, 3d, and 4 were answered in the affirmative, the child would meet the criteria for Oppositional Defiant Disorder, because there was a minimum of one endorsement each for four questions.

Conduct Disorder. Conduct Disorder requires the endorsement of three or more symptoms, at least one of which must have occurred in the past 6 months. In this section, it is particularly important to note that most behaviors must occur more than once to meet criteria. This requirement prevents the diagnosis from being based on a child's experimentation with forbidden behaviors, and focuses instead on the child who is more intent on performing these behaviors. A single instance of a behavior may be scored if it appears unusually severe. For example, a child who, in response to the question "Have you ever set things on fire that you weren't supposed to (for example, trash cans, things at home, clothing, or an animal)," reports setting a fire that injures people or destroys a house would meet this criterion after only a single instance of the behavior.

The interviewer must complete Questions 1–13 before the decision to skip to the next disorder can be made. Even if it feels awkward to ask some children these questions, it *is* necessary to do so. Although a child may have a negative reaction to a question (such as "I would never do anything like that!" or "What kind of a person would hurt an animal?"), asking the question will generally neither cause the child undue distress nor act as a prompt to the child to engage in that behavior. The interviewer can remind the child at this time, "Remember, I told you some questions might fit you pretty well and others won't fit you at all. I just have to do a thorough job. Thanks for being patient with me."

This section also provides criteria for determining whether the disorder, if present, began in Childhood or Adolescence and whether the symptoms are Mild, Moderate, or Severe.

Substance Abuse.   The section covering Substance Abuse is brief and straightforward. Extra space on the scoring form is provided for elaboration of the child's responses. For the purposes of this screening interview, any substance use with resulting impairment is considered to be Substance Abuse. The determination of abuse can be difficult. For example, a child who has had only occasional sips of beer, in the presence of his or her parents, would not meet criteria for this disorder. A child who openly gets drunk *with* his or her parents *would* meet criteria, however, and the interviewer would want to note the circumstances to report to the clinician.

Specific Phobia.   Specific Phobia requires four symptoms to be endorsed. It is very important that the interviewer establish that the child is *very* afraid of the phobic stimulus before counting this symptom as positive. This is crucial because normal fears, even fears of dogs, the dark, and so forth, may be easily overcome by the child in the presence of the stimulus and therefore do not meet criteria for phobia. It is also important that interference with the child's normal routine (Question 4) is present.

> 4. a) **Does your fear of [__] keep you from doing what you would normally do, like . . .** (use appropriate examples, and have child explain answer)
>   i)   **going to sleep at night?**
>   ii)   **going to school or doing your schoolwork?**
>   iii) **playing or going to an activity?**
>   iv)   **doing anything else?**
>   If yes to any, go to 5.

It is *very* important that the child understand this question and answer it appropriately. As stated in the question, the interviewer should have the child explain how the fear interferes with his or her normal activities to confirm that the interviewer and the child are in agreement. Finally, many children will provide examples of something they are afraid of that is developmentally appropriate (e.g., a 6-year-old who still sleeps, without difficulty, using a night light; a 9-year-old who reports being on edge if left alone in the house for several hours at a time). These should not be considered examples of phobic behavior.

At the end of this section, the interviewer is asked to categorize the fear type(s) as Animal, Natural Environment, Blood–Injection–Injury, Situational, and/or Other.

Social Phobia.   Social Phobia requires four symptoms to be endorsed. Again, it is important to differentiate "normal" amounts of stage fright or jitters from a clinical degree of anxiety.

Separation Anxiety Disorder.   Separation Anxiety Disorder requires three or more symptoms to be endorsed. This section focuses on the child's fear of separation from parents. A provision is made for substitution of the child's primary caretaker in cases where the child's parents are not his or her primary caretakers. The correct choice of words is important, because the essence of the disorder is separation from the parental figure. Whether that person is actually the child's parent is not relevant

Particular attention must be paid to the note at the end of Question 4b:

4. a) **Is it hard to go to school because you worry about being away from your parents?** If yes, go to 5.

    b) **Do you often refuse to go to school?** If yes: **Is it because you worry about what will happen to you or your parents while you are gone?** (Score only if both are +.)

In order for Question 4b to count as a symptom of Separation Anxiety Disorder, the child must have school refusal *because* he or she is worried about his or her parents (not, for example, because the child prefers to skip school or cut classes with his or her friends).

Generalized Anxiety Disorder.   The note that appears at the beginning of this section is important:

> **Note:**   If child is positive for Separation Anxiety Disorder, Specific Phobia, or Social Phobia, anxious feelings expressed in this section must be *in addition to* those conditions.

If the child has met criteria for a phobic disorder or for Separation Anxiety Disorder, it is important that he or she not be counted as meeting criteria for Generalized Anxiety Disorder because of the anxiety evidenced in the other disorders. For example, a child who has met criteria for Separation Anxiety Disorder may respond affirmatively to the first question in the Generalized Anxiety Disorder section:

1. **Do you worry more than other kids your age (for example, about things coming up in the future such as starting school, little mistakes you made in the past, taking a test, or seeing the dentist)?** If yes: **Do you worry as often as every day or every other day?** If yes to both, mark box and ask: **What do you worry about?** Record response.

If this occurs, the interviewer should ask the child to provide examples to ensure that the content of the worry is not limited to separation from the primary caretaker but extends to other, unrelated events.

Obsessive-Compulsive Disorder.   In addition to positive responses to Questions 1 and 2 in Section A and/or Questions 1 and 2 in Section B, Obsessive-Compulsive Disorder requires one positive response in Section C. Note that the child must provide examples of obsessions (Section B, Question 1a) and/or compulsions (Section A, Questions 1 and 2) to fulfill criteria. The instruction that "thoughts must be nonsensical, not just excessive 'real-life' worries" reminds the interviewer to differentiate true obsessional thinking from anxious ruminations. The example of compulsions ("like checking, touching, counting, saying, or washing things over and over again") helps the interviewer to differentiate tics or nervous habits (e.g., nail biting, hair twirling) from actual compulsive behaviors.

Stress Disorders.   Both Acute Stress Disorder and Posttraumatic Stress Disorder are contained in this section. For both disorders, the scoring criteria are complex, and familiarity with them is essential for accuracy. A traumatic event must have occurred within the past 4 weeks in order to ask the questions in Section B. Section B must be endorsed in order to diagnose Acute Stress Disorder. Of note, Section D provides for a skip after three symptoms have been endorsed. The end of the Stress Disorders section provides Type criteria for Posttraumatic Stress Disorder: whether the condition is Acute or Chronic, and whether onset was Regular or Delayed.

Eating Disorders.   Anorexia requires one endorsement in each of the first four questions. It should be noted that *both* questions in 1a must be positive in order for 1a to be counted as positive:

1. a) **Have you ever lost weight by putting yourself on a diet or eating different foods than the rest of your family?** If yes: **Did you lose so much weight that someone got worried about you?** (Both must be + to score.) If yes, go to 2.

The purpose of Question 2 is to differentiate normal dieters from individuals who are truly anorectic. If the child is not *currently* too thin (2a), continue with 2b to establish a record of how thin he or she has been. Question 5 is optional and should be asked *only* of girls who are possibly or clearly pubescent.

Bulimia requires one endorsement each Questions 1–4. Note that for this disorder, binges must have occurred at least twice a week for 3 months.

Depression/Dysthymia.   Because these two diagnoses share most symptoms, they are reviewed together. It is important to note the Duration criteria differences. Also, it is important to note when to continue asking a child questions and when to skip to the next section. For example:

1. a) **Have you been feeling sad or depressed [unhappy, low, down in the dumps, crying, moody, miserable]?** If yes, ask:
    b) **Is that happening almost every day?**
    c) **Does that last most of the day?**

All questions should be asked if a child is suspected of suffering from depression, even if all questions in Sections A and B are answered in the negative. Signs to which interviewers need to attend include lack of eye contact, sad appearance, and inability to give a convincing answer to the question about fun activities. For example, a child may answer Question B1a with activities not readily or frequently available (e.g., the only fun activity mentioned is going to Disney World).

Special attention should be given to questions in Section E:

Section E: Psychomotor Changes (Note: Interviewer must confirm this section by observation.)

1. **When you feel [__],**
    a) **do you find that you can't sit still?** (If yes, clarify that this is an increase from baseline.) If yes, go to Section F.
    b) **do you have to keep moving and can't stop?** (If yes, clarify that this is an increase from baseline.) If yes, go to Section F.
    c) **do you wring your hands?** If yes, go to Section F.
    d) **do you pull or rub your clothes, hair, skin, or anything else?** If yes, go to Section F.

If the child responds in the affirmative to these questions, the interviewer must have observed the behavior at some point during the interview in order to score Question 1 as positive. The interviewer should also score this question as positive if he or she observes the behavior during the interview, even if the child denies it. The interviewer must clarify, however, whether the agitation observed is more than that typically displayed by the child (e.g., if he or she has ADHD).

Similarly, impaired concentration (Section H) "counts" as a symptom of depression only if it reflects a *change* in function from baseline (e.g., a child with poor attentional capacity secondary to ADHD must experience deterioration from his or her already low level of attentional capacity in order for the interviewer to score this question as positive).

- *Morbid/Suicidal Thoughts.*   The questions in Section J should always be asked, regardless of whether the child reports a depressed mood or loss of interest. Doing so permits a routine screen for suicide risk in all interviewees.

Mania/Hypomania.   Scoring criteria for these disorders are complex. If irritable mood (Question 2) rather than euphoric/expansive/elated mood (Question 1) is endorsed, four rather than three symptoms in Section B must be endorsed. Interviewers need to be very careful to clarify that a child's positive responses represent truly extraordinary behavior and not the normal fluctuation in activity level experienced by most children. Examples should be provided for any symptom endorsements in Section A.

Enuresis and Encopresis.   The interviewer may be uncomfortable at first in asking some children these questions. If the child is particularly shy or easily embarrassed, it may be wise to preface the section with a statement such as "These next few questions may seem kind of embarrassing or silly, but please bear with me. We're almost done!" Indicate whether enuresis is Nocturnal, Diurnal, or Both.

Note that Enuresis and Encopresis share a single column on the scoring form. Always proceed to Encopresis, even if Enuresis is not endorsed.

Schizophrenia/Psychosis. Again, children may be surprised by the nature of these questions. It may be helpful to say something like, "For some kids, these really are a problem, and I just need to make sure I don't miss anything or skip any questions with you." It is also important to remember the probe at the beginning of this section that asks the interviewer to ascertain whether a response is "real or make-believe." For all real affirmative answers, the interviewer should have the child describe his or her experience.

Three items in Section A deserve special attention:

3. Score if incoherence or marked loosening of associations has been observed during the interview.
4. Score if grossly disorganized or catatonic behavior has been observed.
5. Score if flat or grossly inappropriate affect or an inability (not unwillingness) to speak or an inability to complete any action has been observed during the interview.

These three items require the interviewer to assess the child's behavior during the interview. If such behavior results in discontinuation of the interview, these items should be checked. Most likely, children who have made it this far in the interview will not receive an endorsement for these questions. Examples of positive responses appear below.

- *Incoherence or marked loosening of associations:* Score this as positive if the child has not been able to respond to the interviewer in a consistently meaningful way. Incoherence is exemplified by the child who speaks in sentences composed of words that do not belong together or that are stated or phrased as sentences that have no meaning. The child who frequently and extensively wanders from one topic to another and is difficult for the interviewer to follow is exhibiting loose associations. Many children exhibit these behaviors to a limited degree; thus, Question 3 should be scored only if the child carries the behaviors to an extreme.

- *Grossly disorganized or catatonic behavior:* Catatonic behavior is exemplified by a child who does not move, stares off into space, and appears not to react or interact with his or her surroundings.

- *Flat or grossly inappropriate affect:* Score this as positive if the child exhibited no differential affect at all during the interview, was "blank" and did not react to positive or negative events (flat affect), or expressed emotion not congruent with the topic being discussed (grossly inappropriate affect). *Note:* Many children may demonstrate such behavior to a limited extent (e.g., children sometimes laugh when they are embarrassed). Usually this expression can be redirected to something more appropriate. If it cannot, and if it appears considerably out of proportion to the topic, it may be considered grossly inappropriate.

Psychosocial Stressors. All numbered questions need to be asked of every child. If a child volunteers information concerning any of these questions (especially in the area of physical or sexual abuse), the interviewer should record that information. Probing is not necessary; further probing will be done by a clinician. If the child answers in the affirmative to any of the questions relating to physical or sexual abuse, the interviewer must inform the supervising clinician that there is a need to assess the child's current risk of abuse.

Step 4. Observation of Live Interviews and Videotapes

Following the review of specific disorders, trainees watch a minimum of two demonstration interviews live or on videotape in which the ChIPS is administered by a trained interviewer. Trainees should follow along with the demonstration interview and complete their scoring forms. They should place a slash in boxes for questions they believe have been answered affirmatively and should circle boxes for questions believed to have been answered negatively. In addition, if there are times when the trainee would have continued asking questions, he or she should indicate this by drawing a downward arrow in the box. Similarly, in cases where the trainee would have skipped to the next disorder but the demonstration interviewer continues, he or she should indicate this by drawing a downward arrow with a slash through it in the box. Completed practice scoring forms should then be compared with the demonstration scoring form. Interrater reliability must be at least .90 to be considered adequate.

Next, the trainer should view a training videotape with the group in training, stopping it at least once per syndrome to ask the group what the appropriate response would have been had the child given a different answer. The purpose of this step of training is to provide an efficient way for trainees to obtain a simulated experience with a variety of possible responses.

Step 5. Supervised In Vivo Practice

Conducting interviews under supervision is the final step in training. First, trainees are asked to conduct simulated interviews with each other, with other volunteers, or both. Interviewees should be instructed to make up answers to the questions, and should be encouraged to pretend that they have a certain disorder. This serves several purposes. First, it affords the trainee an opportunity to practice the interview, including the branching (i.e., skip or continue) instructions. Second, being interviewed (as a "child") provides trainees with increased awareness of the interview process and the importance of nonspecific factors in conducting a reliable and valid interview (e.g., the interviewer appearing genuinely interested, appropriately tracking responses, and maintaining an adequate pace). Third, because bogus answers are specified, confidentiality of the interviewee is preserved.

Finally, trainees should administer the ChIPS under real conditions while being observed by a trained interviewer. The purpose of this step is to ensure that the trainee can meet the practical demands of ChIPS administration while simultaneously dealing appropriately with the child. Having an experienced interviewer present also serves as a safeguard or backup in case the trainee has problems during the interview, because that individual is available for consultation. Ideally, one of these first interviews should be videotaped so the trainee and trainer can review the tape together to spot trouble areas or potential problems. It is highly recommended that occasional observation by a trained interviewer occur to prevent administration errors from developing.

Areas of Possible Error in ChIPS Administration

Branching-format errors.   The first area of possible administrator error concerns improper use of the ChIPS branching format. It is critical that interviewers understand the appropriate branching rules for each disorder. Also, when the interviewer has reason to suspect that a disorder is present, continuation of the section would be appropriate. For example, if a child did not answer yes to the first three questions in the Generalized Anxiety Disorder section (1, 2a, and 2b) but had previously indicated other symptoms of anxiety (either verbally or behaviorally), such as worrying about school or worrying about whether he or she was giving the correct answers to questions during the interview, continuation would be appropriate. Continuation would also be appropriate if the child "looked" anxious or if available information indicated that anxiety was a referral question. In these cases, the interviewer should finish the Generalized Anxiety Disorder section; if other positive responses are elicited, the interviewer should return to the initial questions and reask them.

Comprehension errors.   The second area of possible error concerns the process of rephrasing a question when the child does not appear to understand the original wording. There are two basic ways of addressing this problem. First, the child should be instructed at the beginning of the interview to notify the interviewer if he or she does not understand a word or a question. Question 1a from the Oppositional Defiant Disorder section provides an example.

> *Example from Oppositional Defiant Disorder section:*
> I: **Do you usually get upset and lose your temper if things don't go your way?**
> C: What do you mean, "lose my temper"?
> I: It means getting super, super angry. Does that happen to you?
> C: Yeah.

Second, the interviewer should not rely exclusively on the child's requesting clarification. Some children are too embarrassed to admit that they don't know or understand something, and others may simply forget to request clarification from the interviewer. The interviewer must be alert to signals such as the child's nonverbal behavior (e.g., quizzical looks, distracted behavior) and apparently random answers. The interviewer also should be aware that children who have trouble understanding at the beginning of an interview may need to be questioned periodically to ensure that they are, in fact, comprehending the interview as it progresses. A child who indicates a lack of understanding should be praised for being forthright. Under *no* circumstances should a child be criticized for such behavior.

Elaboration errors.   The ChIPS provides examples of allowable clarifications for many questions, such as the following:

> *Example from Conduct Disorder section:*
>
> 12. **Have you ever damaged any property (such as breaking windows, scratching up a car, slashing tires or seats on buses)?**

In this example, the word *property* may appear ambiguous to a child. By providing concrete examples, the question can be clarified. At times, it may be necessary for interviewers to come up with explanations in addition to those provided in the ChIPS. These should be as simple and brief as possible. It may help to find out whether there is a particular word that the child does not understand, such as the word *property* in the example above. If the wording of the question is not the problem, it may help to break the question down into its component parts, as sentence length may be confusing the child.

> *Example from Obsessive-Compulsive Disorder section:*
>
> 1. a) **Do you have bothersome ideas or thoughts that keep coming back into your mind over and over again (like thinking your hands have germs on them, or that you will harm someone, or that things have to be perfectly even)?** If yes, have child describe (thoughts must be nonsensical, not just excessive "real life" worries). If +, go to 2.

If confusion is apparent, this could be rephrased:

> I: Do you have bothersome ideas or thoughts?
> C: Like what?
> I: Like thinking your hands have germs on them, or that you will harm someone, or that things have to be perfectly even?
> C: Yeah.
> I: Do they keep coming back into your mind over and over again?
> C: Yeah.
> I: Could you describe them for me?
> C: (Proceeds with description of troublesome thoughts.)

When the interviewer has completed an explanation, he or she should verify that the child has understood the explanation. A simple "Do you understand?" or "Did that make sense?" may suffice; however, it may also be useful to have the child give an example of what an affirmative response would mean.

Summary

The ChIPS provides an efficient way of collecting standardized diagnostic information from children. The best way to ensure the accuracy, reliability, and validity of the information collected is to adhere to a strict training program for all who use the interview. Necessary steps in training for this interview are as follows:

1. Familiarization with this manual, the instrument, and the scoring materials, as well as a review of childhood psychopathology

2. Group discussion and/or individual tutorial regarding general interviewing procedures with children

3. Group discussion and/or individual tutorial regarding specific details of ChIPS administration, including careful review of the instrument, the scoring form, and the manual on a syndrome-by-syndrome basis

4. Observation of two or more live or videotaped interviews by experienced interviewers

5. Administration of the interview under supervision until satisfactory reliability is obtained

Training interviewers in this manner should increase the reliability of the information gathered with the ChIPS.

References

Achenbach TM: Developmental Psychology: Concepts, Strategies, Methods. New York, Free Press, 1982

American Psychiatric Association: Diagnostic and Statistical Manual: Mental Disorders. Washington, DC, American Psychiatric Association, 1952

American Psychiatric Association: Diagnostic and Statistical Manual of Mental Disorders, 2nd Edition. Washington, DC, American Psychiatric Association, 1968

American Psychiatric Association: Diagnostic and Statistical Manual of Mental Disorders, 3rd Edition. Washington, DC, American Psychiatric Association, 1980

American Psychiatric Association: Diagnostic and Statistical Manual of Mental Disorders, 3rd Edition, Revised. Washington, DC, American Psychiatric Association, 1987

American Psychiatric Association: Diagnostic and Statistical Manual of Mental Disorders, 4th Edition. Washington, DC, American Psychiatric Association, 1994

American Psychological Association: Standards for Educational and Psychological Testing. Washington, DC, American Psychological Association, 1985

Breton JJ, Bergeron L, Valla JP, et al: Do children aged 9 through 11 years understand the DISC version 2.25 questions? J Am Acad Child Adolesc Psychiatry 34:946–954, 1995

Cantwell DP: Classification of childhood and adolescent disorders, in Handbook of Clinical Assessment of Children and Adolescents, Vol 1. Edited by Kestenbaum CJ, Williams DT. New York, New York University Press, 1988, pp 3–18

Chambers WJ, Puig-Antich J, Hirsch M, et al: The assessment of affective disorders in children and adolescents by semi-structured interview. Arch Gen Psychiatry 42:696–702, 1985

Costello AJ, Edelbrock C, Kalas R, Kessler MD, Klaric S: The NIMH Diagnostic Interview Schedule for Children (DISC). Unpublished manuscript, Western Psychiatric Institute and Clinic, Pittsburgh, PA, 1982

Edelbrock C, Costello AJ: Structured psychiatric interviews for children and adolescents, in Handbook of Psychological Assessment. Edited by Goldstein G, Hersen M. New York, Pergamon, 1984, pp 276–290

Edelbrock C, Costello AJ, Dulcan MK, et al: Parent–child agreement on child psychiatric symptoms assessed via structured interview. Journal of Psychological Psychiatry 27:181–190, 1986

Fristad MA, Emery BL, Beck SJ: Use and abuse of the Children's Depression Inventory. J Consult Clin Psychol 65:699–702, 1997

Fristad MA, Teare M, Weller EB, et al: Study III: development and concurrent validity of the Children's Interview for Psychiatric Syndromes—Parent Version (P-ChIPS). J Child Adolesc Psychopharmacol 8:219–224, 1998a

Fristad MA, Cummins J, Verducci JS, et al: Study IV: concurrent validity of the DSM-IV–revised Children's Interview for Psychiatric Syndromes (ChIPS). J Child Adolesc Psychopharmacol 8:227–236, 1998b

Fristad MA, Glickman AR, Verducci JS, et al: Study V: Children's Interview for Psychiatric Syndromes (ChIPS): psychometrics in two community samples. J Child Adolesc Psychopharmacol 8:237–245, 1998c

Harris JR, Liebert RM: The Child: Development From Birth to Adolescence, 2nd Edition. Englewood Cliffs, NJ, Prentice-Hall, 1987, p 370

Helzer JE: The use of a structured diagnostic interview for routine psychiatric evaluations. J Nerv Ment Dis 169:45–49, 1981

Herjanic B, Reich W: Development of a structured psychiatric interview for children: agreement between parent and child on individual symptoms. J Abnorm Child Psychol 10:307–324, 1982

Herjanic B, Herjanic M, Brown F, et al: Are children reliable reporters? J Abnorm Child Psychol 3:41–48, 1975

Hetherington EM, Martin B: Family factors and psychopathology in children, in Psychopathological Disorders of Childhood, 3rd Edition. Edited by Quay HC, Werry JS. New York, John Wiley & Sons, 1979, pp 332–390

Hodges K, Kline J, Stern L, et al: The development of a child assessment interview for research and clinical use. J Abnorm Psychol 10:173–189, 1982

Jaynes S, Charles E, Kass F, et al: Clinical supervision of the initial interview: effects on patient care. Am J Psychiatry 136:1454–1457, 1979

Kessler JW: Nosology in child psychopathology, in Perspectives in Child Psychopathology. Edited by Rie HE. Chicago, IL, Aldine-Atherton, 1971, pp 85–129

Kovacs M: The Interview Schedule for Children (ISC). Psychopharmacol Bull 21:991–994, 1985

Lapouse R, Monk MA: An epidemiologic study of behavior characteristics of children. Am J Public Health 48:1134–1144, 1958

Maier HW: Three Theories of Child Development. New York, Harper & Row, 1965

Othmer E, Penick EC, Powell BJ, et al: Psychiatric Diagnostic Interview (PDI). Los Angeles, CA, Western Psychological Services, 1981

Puig-Antich J, Chambers W: The Schedule for Affective Disorders and Schizophrenia for School-Aged Children (Kiddie-SADS). New York, New York State Psychiatric Institute, 1978

Reich W, Welner Z: Diagnostic Interview for Children and Adolescents, DSM-III-R Version (DICA-R-C). Unpublished manuscript, Washington University, Division of Child Psychiatry, St. Louis, MO, 1988

Robins LN: Epidemiology: reflections on testing the validity of psychiatric interviews. Arch Gen Psychiatry 42:918–924, 1985

Rutter M, Graham P: The reliability and validity of the psychiatric assessment of the child, I: interview with the child. Br J Psychiatry 114:565–579, 1968

Shaffer D, Fisher P, Piacentini J, et al: Diagnostic Interview Schedule for Children (DISC-2.25)—Child Version—Parent Version. New York, New York State Psychiatric Institute, Division of Child and Adolescent Psychiatry, 1991

Stevenson GS, Smith G: Child Guidance Clinics: A Quarter Century of Development. New York, Commonwealth Fund, 1934

Teare M, Fristad MA, Weller EB, et al: Study I: Development and criterion validity of the Children's Interview for Psychiatric Syndromes (ChIPS). J Child Adolesc Psychopharmacol 8:205–211, 1998a

Teare M, Fristad MA, Weller EB, et al: Study II: Concurrent validity of the DSM-III-R Children's Interview for Psychiatric Syndromes (ChIPS). J Child Adolesc Psychopharmacol 8:213–219, 1998b

Verducci JS, Mack ME, DeGroot MH: Estimating multiple rater agreement for a rare diagnosis. Journal of Multivariate Analysis 27:512–535, 1988

Weller EB, Weller RA, Teare M, Fristad MA: Children's Interview for Psychiatric Syndromes (ChIPS). Unpublished manuscript, University of Kansas School of Medicine, Department of Child Psychiatry, Kansas City, KS, October 1985

Yule W: The epidemiology of child psychopathology, in Advances in Clinical Child Psychology, Vol 4. Edited by Kazdin AE, Lahey BB. New York, Plenum, 1981